CREATE YOUR OWN MAGIC FOR CLNC® SUCCESS

SECOND EDITION

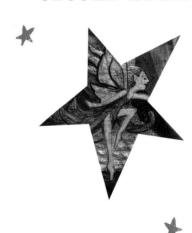

Other Books and Programs by
Vickie L. Milazzo, RN, MSN, JD

CLNC® Certification Program
(Seminar, DVD and Audio CD)

NACLNC® and Private Apprenticeships
(Seminar, DVD and Audio CD)

CLNC® Success Stories, Third Edition (editor)

Core Curriculum for Legal Nurse Consulting® Textbook, 13ᵗʰ Edition

I Am a Successful CLNC® Success Journal

Flash 55 Promotions: 55 Free Ways to Promote Your CLNC® Business, Second Edition

Legal Nurse Consulting Ezine (editor)

101 Great Ways to Improve Your Life (coauthor)

Rising to the Top—A Guide to Self-Development (coauthor)

Roadmap to Success (coauthor)

Wall Street Journal Bestseller
Inside Every Woman: Using the 10 Strengths You Didn't Know You Had to Get the Career and Life You Want Now

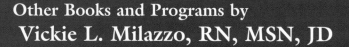

Vickie Milazzo Institute™
National Alliance of Certified Legal Nurse Consultants

CREATE YOUR OWN MAGIC FOR CLNC® SUCCESS

SECOND EDITION

A UNIQUE BOOK OF 91 DEVILISHLY PRACTICAL POTIONS

Vickie L. Milazzo, RN, MSN, JD

THE PIONEER OF LEGAL NURSE CONSULTING

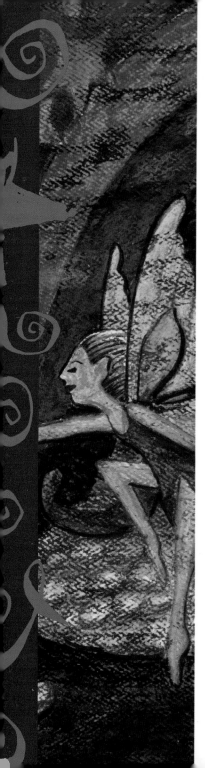

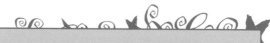

To my husband Tom,
the magic of my life.

CREATE YOUR OWN MAGIC
FOR CLNC® SUCCESS
SECOND EDITION

ISBN-13: 978-1-933216-62-1
ISBN-10: 1-933216-62-X

Publisher: Vickie Milazzo Institute, a division of
Medical-Legal Consulting Institute, Inc.
5615 Kirby Drive, Suite 425
Houston, Texas 77005-2448
713.942.2200
LegalNurse.com

First printing, March 2003
Second printing, April 2005
Third printing, June 2008

Printed in the United States of America.
Printed on acid free paper (∞).

Contents

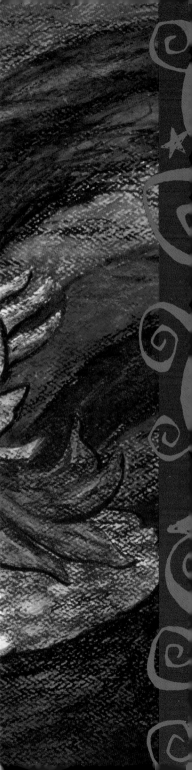

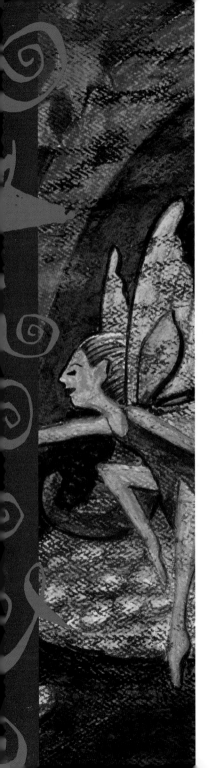

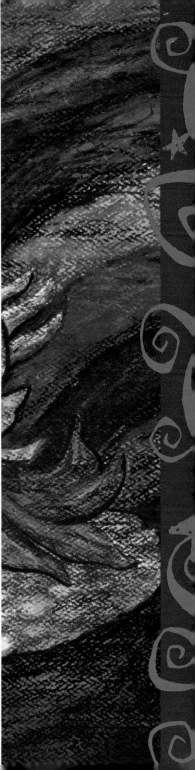

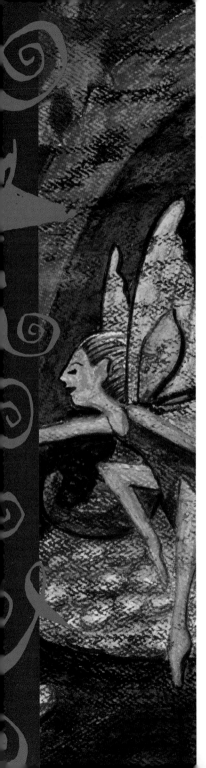

Introduction

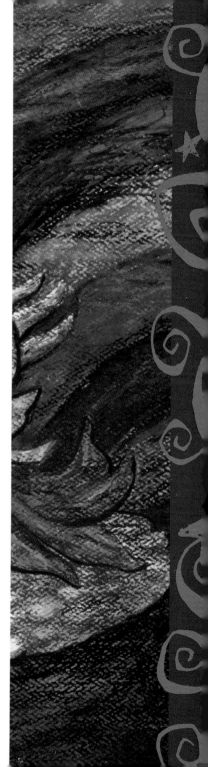

I nside each of us lies a desire to do something spectacular—to fly, to write, to sculpt, to climb mountains or perhaps to step off into the unknown and create a business where none existed. That space between vision and creation is a magical land filled with wondrous adventure but also with treacherous pathways and fierce, fire-breathing dragons.

Maneuvering in such a land requires that we suspend fear and embrace valor. Yet courage alone is not enough. A courageous fool is no less a fool.

With the tools, skills and knowledge to conquer the unknown, we shape our own destiny, we forge a new reality. We reach to the stars and grasp handfuls of wonder.

When I stepped out for my own adventure in 1982, I had no guidebook. I pioneered the field of legal nurse consulting, carving a new industry in an uncharted land, conquering the dragons and narrowly skirting the pitfalls. What I did have was vision, persistence and the voices of my favorite inspirational coaches urging me onward and upward.

I found those coaches in books and audio CDs, in seminars and conferences and in the people who really believed in me. While they gave no specific direction for my own vision, they nevertheless guided me with encouragement and general insights. They lifted me when I stumbled. They gave me a mental high-five when I reached a goal. And when the shadows and fears closed in on me, my coaches could usually make me laugh away the darkness.

In writing *Create Your Own Magic for CLNC® Success,* my goal is to shine some starlight onto your path into the magical world of business and entrepreneurship. I would especially like to acknowledge the team at Vickie Milazzo Institute who helped bring this book to creation and three people, Leigh Owen, Chris Rogers and Roxann Combs, who surely have some wizard in them.

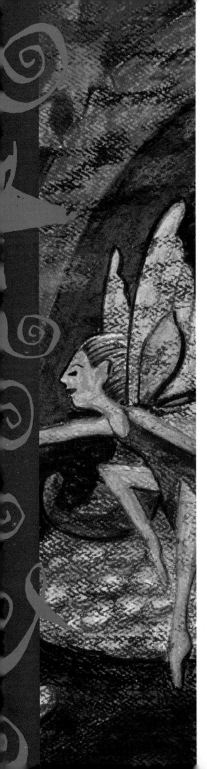

How to Use this CLNC® Success Book of 91 Magic Potions

As you read, you will don the hat of the wizard that you must surely become and discover the spells of transformation. You will discover that the lightest elixirs of laughter and joy are just as important as the most powerful enchantments of hard work and determination. Within these pages you will find everything you need to take that first shaky step, to maneuver among the dragons and to enjoy the glory of success—all presented in a lighthearted, easy-to-use manner.

Begin by reading this book of potions as you would explore a treasure chest. Browse. Sample. Enjoy. Then don your sorcerer's hat, and flip these pages until one special magical potion speaks to you. Merlin the wizard assures me this is the potion you should conjure first. Focus on it for seven days, taking one action step each day.

Create Your Own Magic for CLNC® Success provides the pixie dust to power your magic carpet. Hop on, hold tight and enjoy an incredible success journey.

1. Write your CLNC® success story. Be vivid. For example: What year is it? What does your office look like? Where is it located? How many attorney-clients do you have? How much are your revenues? How are you enjoying your new financial prosperity?

2. Complete the magical potion in the book that promises the most impact in helping you achieve your CLNC® success story.

3. Then complete the next potion. Then the next.

4. Expose yourself to a new idea each day or each week. Earmark the ideas that stretch your imagination and revisit them again and again.

5. To make each potion your own, expand and rewrite the recipes, adding your own magical ingredients that no other CLNC® wizard can duplicate. Make them work for you.

Chances are you have other business books on your shelf—deep, darkly instructive and perhaps dusty. You'll find this one entirely different. It's a friendly book, fun to read yet highly instructive. Anytime you question your vision or your pathway, dip into the pages and you'll find a magic spell to guide you in those next enchantingly frightful steps of becoming a most successful CLNC® professional.

Your CLNC® Master Wizard,

Vickie

Vickie L. Milazzo, RN, MSN, JD

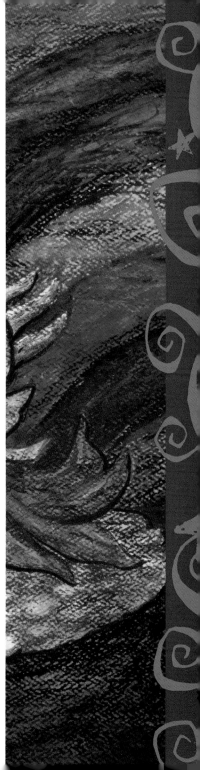

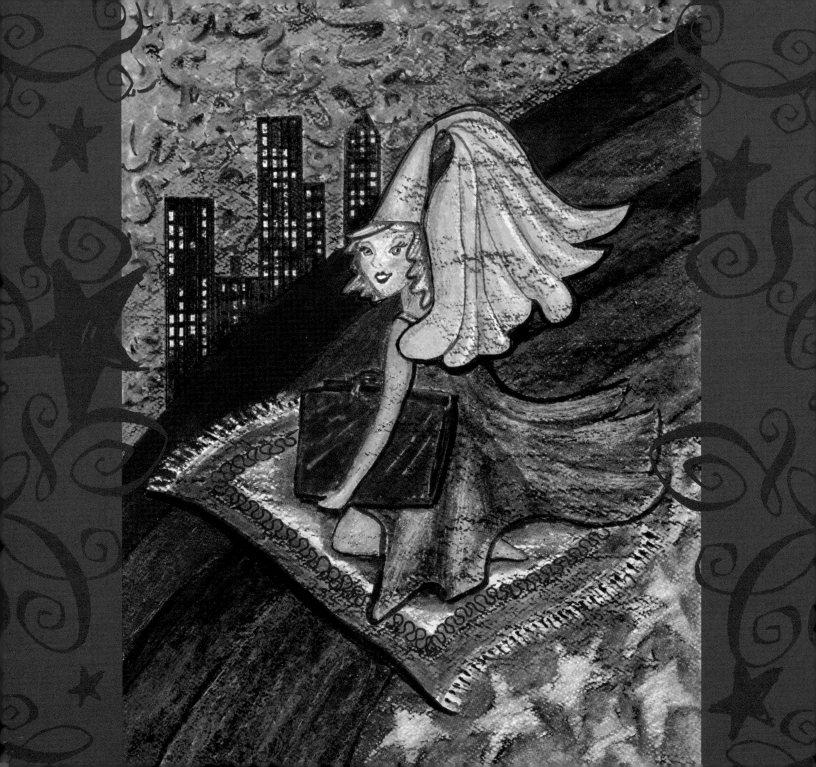

Launch Your CLNC® Magic Carpet Ride

Every wizard of entrepreneurship must possess four talismans—a passionate vision, a star-studded plan, action to move the plan forward and the enthusiastic persistence to live and enjoy your vision each day. With these four talismans and the magic spells, potions and hexes you'll discover on the following pages, you will artfully fly through tough situations and capture the pixie spirits that favor success.

Using these spells and potions, you'll ignite your passion, embrace audacious goals and grow a dazzlingly successful business.

You'll experience the exhilarating high of building your CLNC® magic kingdom, and you'll gain rewards far beyond worldly revenue. You'll create a marketing strategy, a business plan and a timeline for CLNC® success.

You'll grow from conjurer to Master Wizard in a devilishly short time. You'll create your own enchanting magic carpet ride to extraordinary success.

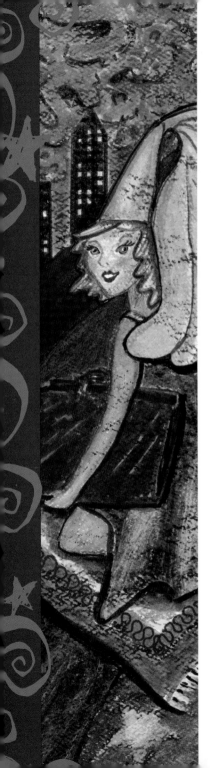

✦ Ignite Your Passion ✦

"Do what you love and you'll never work a day in your life."
— *Confucius*

Conjure a vision: One handyman attacks chores with zeal—practically needs to be restrained from preparatory trips to the hardware store. Others walk the plank to the garage at sword point. One gardener enjoys magical hours weeding, mulching, planting and pruning, while another dutifully mows grass and trims shrubs. The difference in these varied outlooks is *passion*. The passionate enjoyment of your work is the ultimate enchantment. When you invoke the following spell, your hidden passion will burst into view like a rainbow after a rain.

Gather your conjuring tools:

* A pen or pencil and writing paper
* Highlighter markers (your favorite captivating colors)
* A quietly hypnotic location indoors or out
* 15 minutes of uninterrupted time

Optional charm:

Now, Discover Your Strengths
by Marcus Buckingham and Donald Clifton

Stimulate your imagination by spending two minutes jotting down everything that needs to be done this week. Time yourself. Set that list aside.

Take another two minutes to list the things you'd do if you had no obligations and if money were not an issue.

Make a third two-minute list of the long-term goals you want to achieve, including items in the areas of personal relationships, family, friends, health, finance, continuing education, spiritual growth, travel and leisure.

Turn all three lists upside down and pull out a clean sheet of paper.

Imagine you only have one week to live, and you can live that week in good health. In one minute, write down what you would do—what would bring you pure joy—and the people you would want with you during that incredible week. Usually, this last item is an eye opener that puts all else in perspective. You have found your number one priority. This is your passion.

Now, turn over your lists and, with your new-found passion in mind, highlight three priorities on each. Work these into your schedule and do them without fail.

Sorcerer's Suggestion: Discovering your passion is like seeing the rainbow. It's beautiful to look at, but it's out there in the distance. Take action to follow your rainbow to the pot of gold. Open your heart to more fully ignite your passion. Network with other passionate, successful people; model their practices. Find your strengths within that passion and seek opportunities to inspire passion in your daily work.

Gaze into Your Crystal Ball to Become a Visionary

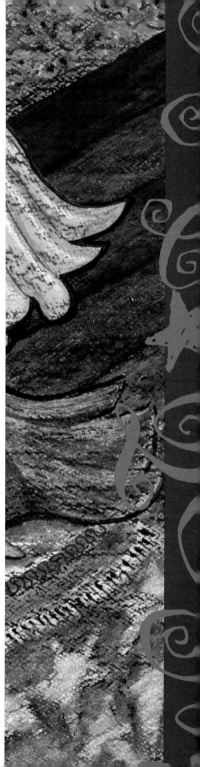

Look into your crystal ball. Where will you be in five years? In ten years? What magic will you use to get there? Who will fly along with you? And why do you want to go? Focus on a vivid, spellbinding vision of your ideal future and you will move toward your success goals with deceptive ease.

Start your magic spell with:

* A charmingly quiet spot—indoors or out—with no clock, no cell phone
* Comfortable conjuring clothes
* Writing paper and colored pens or pencils
* A packet of Post-It® notes
* Pictures or a magazine collage of your goals
* A thesaurus
* Enchanting music
* A measure of time that is ample and specific

Optional elixir:

A goal-setting book such as *Wishcraft: How to Get What You Really Want* **by Barbara Sher and Annie Gotlieb**

Stir your creative mind with a portent: imagine an ideal workday five years in the future. Think about your compelling reason for living.

Continue stirring the brew, adding your personal values, passions and dreams. Write a couple of pages without censoring your ideas. Draw pictures. Keep your pencil moving. Stay in the vision.

When the writing stops—and before you revise what you've written—stand up, stretch and break the spell for a moment.

Then read, distill and polish until you have a single sentence:

My Vision Is_____

_____

> **Wizard's Tip:** Your vision statement is a living document and a bit of fortune telling. Keep it current. Keep it in sight. Read the invocation daily and it will guide you to your magical ideal future.

A sample spell that has worked magic for Vickie Milazzo Institute:
Revolutionizing Nursing Careers One RN at a Time Since 1982

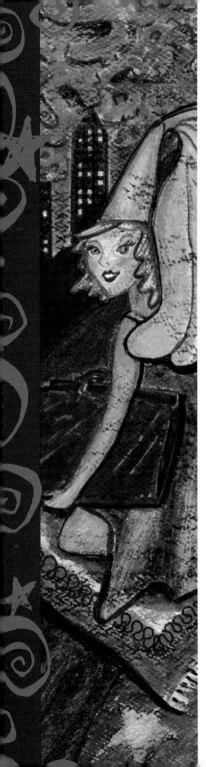

LIVE YOUR CORE VALUES

Aladdin and the selfish Prince Achmed both pursued Princess Jasmine, but Achmed's core values doomed him to failure. Aladdin, armed with such positive values as love, passion and adventure, carried Jasmine on his magic carpet into the star-filled night. When your core values are true to your goals and desires, you are empowered to achieve wondrous results.

Start your crystal gazing with:

* A list of positive values you want to attain
* A list of negative values you want to avoid
* A half hour of uninterrupted time

Optional elixir:

Daily Reflections for Highly Effective People by Stephen R. Covey

Prioritize. Compare the first two values—for example, love and success. Ask yourself: If I could have all the love I want in the world, but no success, or all the success in the world but no love, which would I choose? In the same manner, compare the value you choose to the next in line. Continue all the way down the list of positive values. On the negative list, ask which do I most want to avoid?

Rewrite the two lists in order of priority.

Identify and highlight your top three values in each list.

Compare your priorities. We naturally move toward pleasure and away from pain, toward our positive values and away from the negatives. If your top values are in conflict, then your actions will be conflicting and less effective. If, for example, the top positive value is adventure, but the top negative value is pain, you must overcome a fear of pain to seek adventure.

How do your values support being a successful CLNC® consultant? If any value, such as fun, does not serve you as well right now as another, such as passion, you can intentionally change the priority order and then act accordingly.

My priority values are _____

_____

_____

> **Aladdin's Advice:** Remember that actions speak louder than words. Follow your core values in every part of your life. Remember also that a change in circumstance can change your core values. Review and reprioritize every six months to assure your magic carpet is still flying toward the stars. Finally, remember that you represent the reputation and future of all CLNC® consultants. Be an enchantingly positive influence and a role model in all your professional actions.

Suggested core values

* *Positive*—Love, success, freedom, intimacy, security, adventure, power, passion, comfort, health, fun, integrity (other _____, _____, _____)
* *Negative*—Rejection, anger, frustration, loneliness, depression, failure, pain, burnout, stress, guilt, boredom (other _____, _____, _____)

Ride Your Magic Carpet with Audacious Goals

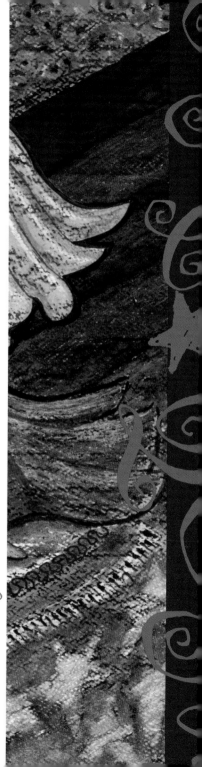

At the end of the rainbow is the pot of gold. If you want the gold, then you must get over the rainbow. Goal-setting is that simple. If you don't set a goal to ride your magic carpet over the rainbow, you'll need more than a captive leprechaun to get your hands on that gold.

Assemble the magical ingredients:

* An enchantingly private location
* Paper, pen and pencil
* Quietly inspirational music or silence
* A half hour of uninterrupted time

Optional elixir:

Goal-setting books or audio CDs

Examine your mind-set. Only 50% of the population is motivated by goals, the other 50% is motivated by problems. Would a coveted prize, such as money, vacation or fame, move you to action? Or would you respond to a problem that needs to be solved, knowing you are the best, most experienced person to tackle it? If you are a problem solver, simply envision your goals as intriguing problems to be solved.

Recognize what is preventing you from making a written plan for achieving goals. Do you fear being pinned down to one road when a better one might present itself at any time? That's okay—write your goals in pencil. Any decision is erasable, and you should periodically review, update and change your goals to match your dreams.

Written goals are proven to be more powerful than unwritten goals. Nevertheless, fewer than three percent of Americans have written goals. You'll be far ahead of the norm by simply writing them down.

Be willing to back into it. If you have difficulty deciding what you want:

* Consider outcomes you *absolutely do not* want. For example, "I do not want to work in a hospital the rest of my life."
* Then write down some short-term compromises that will get you to your rainbow. "I will work in a hospital part time while I build my CLNC® business."
* Finally, ease in to recognizing what you *do* want. "I will be a financially independent full-time Certified Legal Nurse Consultant℠ by _____ (date)."

> **Wizard's Wisdom:** Big, audacious goals will power your magic carpet over the rainbow and into the stars. Write down at least three specific, measurable goals. Project a time for completion. Set intermittent milestones. Make sure your long-term goals are reflected in your daily "to do" list, take action and grab a reward from that pot of gold each time you complete a goal.

Examples of results-oriented goals

* "I will obtain one new attorney-client per month."
* "I will earn $_____ this year."

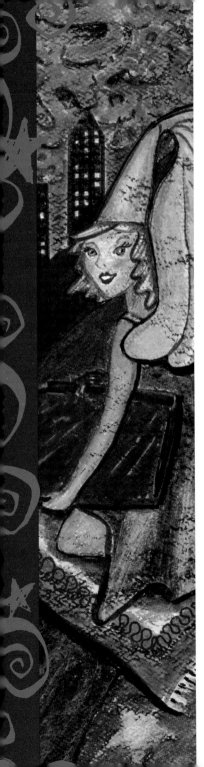

PLAN FOR YOUR SWEET SPELL OF SUCCESS

Your business plan is your personal Excalibur, a magic sword that cuts through the confusion of building a successful CLNC® practice. The sharpest plan is concise and simple. It defines your business goals, objectives and opportunities. It projects revenues, market development, organizational growth and service expansion. Sharpen your sword regularly on the sorcerer's stone of planning and it will gleam with golden brilliance as it points your way.

ASSEMBLE YOUR SORCERER'S TOOLS:

★ Your vision statement—business and personal
★ Your mission statement—business and personal
★ Your business goals—objectives and strategies
★ Your competitive advantage or unique selling position—USP
★ A list of your strengths and weaknesses
★ Your projected budget for business development
★ Your projected operating expenses
★ A one-year calendar

OPTIONAL TALISMAN:

Business plan software or a book such as *Business Plans for Dummies* by Paul Tiffany and Steven D. Peterson

Awaken your clairvoyance by writing a brief essay describing your business one year in the future. Envision yourself at your desk.

• How has your CLNC® business changed?
• How has your revenue grown?
• How have your strengths guided your CLNC® business? What is your market niche and how did you carve that niche?
• Who are your attorney-clients?
• How is your business structured? Which processes are outsourced? Who are the wizards and pixies who keep it running smoothly?
• Which opportunities provided expansion? How did you follow up on those opportunities?

Forecast milestones in the development of your business. Guided by your intuition, and using your calendar and your essay, schedule dates for achieving specific goals.

Merlin's Tip: Even a magical sword needs a keen edge. Keep your CLNC® business plan sharp and it will cleave the way to a fascinating and successful career.

A WIZARD'S ELIXIR

Go to your online NACLNC® Community for CLNC® members only to receive your treasure trove of business development resources, links and recommended list of authoritative textbooks.

TRANSFORM FEARLESSLY FROM APPRENTICE TO CLNC® WIZARD

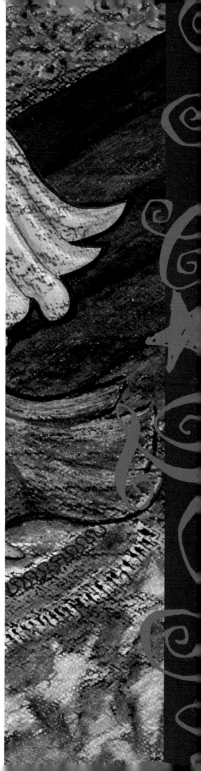

Merlin, Tinkerbell and Cinderella's fairy godmother were all sorcerers' apprentices before they learned to use their powers. As you learn the tricks of your new trade, recognize that, as a powerful wizard of nursing, you are already a virtuoso in the eyes of most attorneys. The transition to CLNC® wizard is as easy as *alakazam!*

Start your magic transformation with:

* A captivating resume that highlights your accomplishments
* A dazzling business card and brochure
* A powerful business presence that exudes confidence, no matter how fluttery you feel inside
* Your magical CLNC® study materials
* The knowledge that mistakes are rarely fatal

Optional elixir:

Affirmations that support your expert status

Practice making your presentation. Practice, practice, practice—perfect practice of interview responses breaks the spell of looking like a beginner.

Study everything you can find about being a CLNC® professional.

Team up with an experienced CLNC® colleague and start your apprenticeship as a CLNC® subcontractor.

Be willing and ready to make and learn from plenty of mistakes.

Create a one-page reminder of your goals and strengths, and read this page every day until you feel confident you've achieved professionalism in your new CLNC® practice.

> **Wizard's Tip:** Don't be intimidated by attorneys or other Certified Legal Nurse Consultants℠. Even experienced CLNC® consultants were once apprentices. You possess your own magic and expertise attorneys need. But don't expect to know everything. Recognize when to call for assistance from a fellow CLNC® wizard or CLNC® subcontractor.

 CLNC® sample affirmations

"I am a successful CLNC® consultant."
"I am a nurse and I can do anything!"

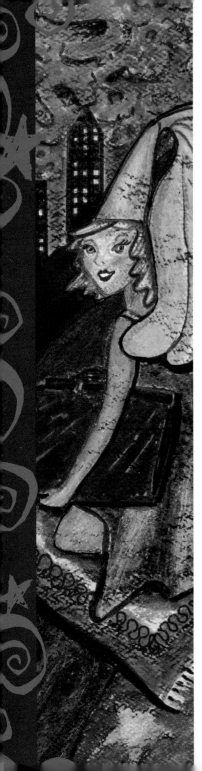

 # Grow a Dazzling CLNC® Practice

Dreamers make the extraordinary happen. By the power of your wizardry and your vision, your CLNC® practice will flourish and expand. You will be sought as an expert, a magus, a wonder-worker, while your behind-the-scenes team keeps the magic lantern burning. To reach your potential, you must think big. Dream big. Imagine the end result, then brew up the hexes, philters and potions that will make that vision materialize on the corporeal plane.

Assemble your alchemist's tools:

- ✷ A captivating vision
- ✷ A dazzling desire
- ✷ A medley of resources
- ✷ A steadfast foundation
- ✷ A dependable organizational structure
- ✷ A spellbinding set of precisely chiseled goals
- ✷ A cup of determination
- ✷ A dash of trust in yourself and others

Optional elixir:

An inspiring book, such as *You'll See It When You Believe It: The Way to Your Personal Transformation* by Wayne W. Dyer or *The E-Myth Revisited: Why Most Small Businesses Don't Work and What to Do About It* by Michael E. Gerber

Invoke your growth plan

This is the time to think like an entrepreneur, not like a technician.

Review your vision and goals and open your mind to new possibilities. Where are you in respect to your original dream? Now it's time to grow your CLNC® practice.

Consider your next step. Diversify by adding new services and attracting new attorney-clients.

Expand your organizational structure, engage CLNC® subcontractors or hire part- or full-time employees to go for larger, more diverse contracts. Alchemy is the art of turning ordinary matter into gold. This could be just the right time to raise your fees, hand off cases to a trusted CLNC® subcontractor or leverage current contracts to higher yield by expanding the CLNC® services you offer your clients.

Think outside the traditional legal nurse consulting culture. Implement a new marketing strategy. Join a CEO group. Get your annual recharge at the *National Alliance of Certified Legal Nurse Consultants* Annual Conference, where you'll learn from and network with Vickie and the most successful CLNC® Pros.

Based on your new vision, cast the runes for new milestones in the areas of advertising, operations, finance and space requirements—and always market, market, market.

> **Wizard's Wisdom:** Consult tea leaves, a crystal ball or a Ouija board—but your own imagination, determination and enthusiasm will more keenly divine your future. Create CLNC® alliances. Schedule a yearly event with your fellow alchemists to brainstorm your company's growth. Commit to constant and never-ending improvement. Learn from your mistakes, practice taking risks and never say never.

A successful Certified Legal Nurse Consultant℠ who worked magic

"While in transition from part time to full time, my legal nurse consulting revenues were $85,000. The next year I hired my first employee and massively exceeded my goal of grossing $200,000. My annual revenue now exceeds $1,000,000."

—*Suzanne E. Arragg,*
RN, BSN, CDONA/LTC, CLNC, California

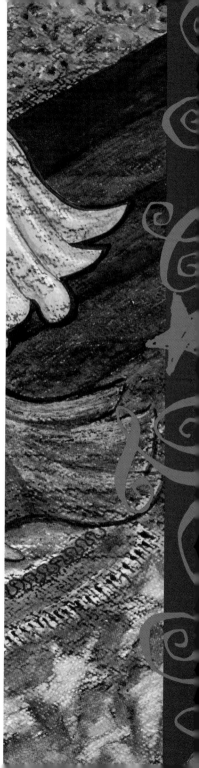

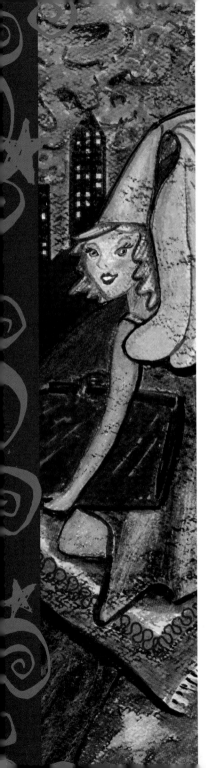

Use CLNC®
Subcontractors to
Build Your Magic Kingdom

"I would rather earn one percent of 100 people's efforts," financial wizard J. Paul Getty once said, "than 100 percent of my own." The wizardry in subcontracting means leveraging other people's time, energy, talents, money, knowledge and effort to achieve your desired goals. Use this spell to achieve your financial goals faster than *presto-chango!*

Start your magic spell with:

✶ An established attorney-client relationship
✶ *NACLNC®* Online Directory
✶ A list of tasks and cases to subcontract
✶ A subcontractor agreement form with a confidentiality clause
✶ A dependable tracking method

Develop a relationship of mutual respect and confidence with attorney-clients, so they trust and appreciate your CLNC® subcontractor pool. You are responsible for assuring quality work product from each of your CLNC® subcontractors.

• Identify CLNC® subcontractors before you urgently need them. Assess their qualifications. Assign a simple conjuration to see how quickly and accurately they respond.
• Match the CLNC® sub to an appropriate assignment.

• Communicate clearly. CLNC® subcontractors must understand their assignments, your deadlines and your established procedures for interacting with and reporting to the attorney.
• Track and evaluate the project's status.

To produce a consistent work product despite having a host of CLNC® subs, use templates for reports, chronologies and screenings.

Enchanter's Sleight-of-Hand: Assign CLNC® subs to cases outside your area of expertise and to do simple projects, such as research and developing chronologies. By effectively delegating and managing the work of excellent CLNC® subs, you expand your kingdom, become more productive and achieve the greatest personal, professional and financial success. The rainbow to the pot of gold is paved with leveraged talent.

Qualities to look for in your CLNC® subcontractors

Dedicated to servicing you and your clients.
Resides outside your geographical area (to avoid competition).
Top-flight nursing and legal nurse consulting skills.
Ability to produce quality work product on time and with minimal supervision.

Exorcise Detours, Bad Ideas and Other Hallucinations

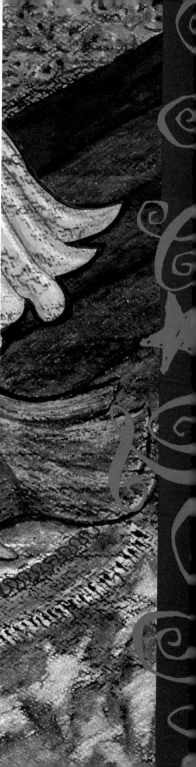

Your magic carpet dips and soars, past intriguing skyscrapers and into the stars. Each star might be an exciting alternate route to the same destination or an alluring sidetrack that takes you off your purpose. How do you know the difference?

Start your spellbinding excursion with:

* Your vision statement
* Your business plan
* Your marketing plan
* Your core values
* Your financial goals

Optional elixir:

An energizing song, such as the CLNC® "National Anthem." It will summon your vision each time you hear it.

Examine the idea by writing out the goal, the obstacles to overcome and the prize to be won if it works as expected.

Review your vision statement. Does this remarkable idea support the vision?

Review your business plan. Is the alluring new idea within the scope of your projected goals?

Review your marketing plan. Will this amazing idea enlarge the projected results without detracting from or sapping energy needed to implement important marketing strategies?

Review your core values.

Review your financial goals. Can this new star be explored without unfavorable drain on your financial resources?

> **Shaman's Tip:** Run the idea by several honest and trusted wizards and be open to their responses. Is it still a good idea? Can you pursue it without throwing your magic carpet out of balance? Remember the four talismans that keep your carpet aloft—a passionate vision, a plan, action to move the plan forward and the enthusiastic persistence to live and enjoy your vision. If your idea is on track, then write it into your business plan, integrate the timeline, delegate resources and pursue it. Be patient, persistent and remain focused. If the stars in your eyes are merely masking an intriguing detour, then abandon the idea, no matter how alluring its promise.

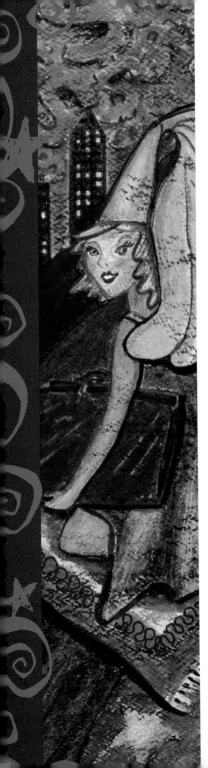

Be a Wizard for Life

A successful wizard doesn't stop learning once the herb tables and transfiguration spells have been memorized. School is never out, because life and business are constantly unfolding. The brain responds to exercise. Using it keeps it strong—and the following spell will ensure mental agility at any age.

Start your incantation with:

✴ Books, audio CDs and business DVDs
✴ A learning plan

Optional elixir:

Inside Every Woman: Using the 10 Strengths You Didn't Know You Had to Get the Career and Life You Want Now by Vickie L. Milazzo

Develop the mindset to feed your brain new knowledge every day. Create a mesmerizing mental gymnasium to strengthen your new muscles. Swap TV, talk radio and computer games for books, CDs and other magical learning instruments that open your mind to powerful new ideas.

Design a learning plan and commit at least 15 minutes a day. Build on present knowledge or expand into new areas of wizardry.

Use short study periods—15 minutes followed by a five-minute break—to boost retention. We retain the most information from the beginning and end of each study period. Breaking two study hours into 15-minute segments provides six times as many opportunities for retention as does a solid two-hour cram.

Find something that excites you personally or professionally about whatever you have to learn. Passion helps us remember.

Break the material down into manageable segments. Apply what you learn. Practice it. If a book has exercises, do them. Share what you learn. Once you teach it to a friend, you own it.

Soothsayer's Secret: Repetition increases retention. Pick a topic you want to learn and study for at least two 15-minute periods every day by reading the material into a recorder. Listen to the recording in your car or while doing boring tasks—washing dishes, jogging, cleaning the garage, sorting laundry or polishing your crystal ball. While your logical mind is busy waxing the broomstick, your creative mind eagerly absorbs the information. You'll be magically exercising both sides of the brain.

A mastermind learning group

Have you ever read a book or listened to a CD and felt tremendously excited about putting that material into practice—only to realize months later that you never took the first step? Combine a mastermind group with a learning plan. Choose a topic you all want to study, decide on a book and work through the book with a group of wizards. Meet weekly or biweekly to discuss each chapter and how you can apply the knowledge. Hold each other to task so the entire group benefits.

Immortalize Your Magic

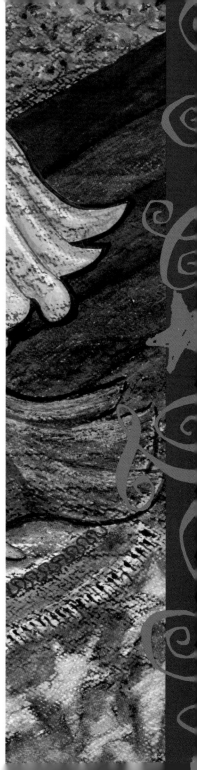

Even the most beautiful silver will tarnish if left unpolished. Yet one swipe of a cloth polishes the lamp and summons the magic genie again. What is that special something that makes your business rewarding and exciting? What motivates you to tackle the tough jobs? Recognize that holding onto the magic of your business adventure means keeping the pixie dust and the polishing tools handy.

Start your magic spell with:

* Upbeat, motivated people
* A captivating journal or scrapbook of your accomplishments
* Spellbinding pictures of your goals
* Newspaper articles and publications related to big cases on which you've worked
* A list of alternating tasks—intense projects and light projects
* Break-time activities
* A list of new skills you want to develop
* A list of extraordinary new services you want to offer
* An active time-keeping system to record your daily earnings

Optional Elixir:

Books and audio CDs by motivational speakers you admire, such as Deepak Chopra, Anthony Robbins, Brian Tracy and Vickie L. Milazzo

Create a motivating work environment by surrounding yourself with reminders of why you began your CLNC® practice. Post pictures of your goals, your family, a favorite vacation spot or a house, car or boat you want to own. Keep a magical scrapbook filled with symbols of your successfully completed milestones—attorney letters, notes, cards, photos, emails, photocopies of your big checks, reminders of your big cases—and browse through the scrapbook frequently. Frame your favorites.

Activate your motivational energy by varying your routine. Alternate mentally intense projects with smaller, easier projects, and reward yourself for a job well done. Take frequent breaks. Get out of the office and spend time smelling the roses. Buy a hammock. Play motivating music.

Meditate often on the big picture. Invest a few minutes each day looking forward to wondrous new enchantments for your business. Great wizards also gaze backward to reflect on the progress they've made. Charge what you're worth. Stay mesmerized by your vision and keep your sense of humor.

Genie's Tip: Associate with winners. Join business organizations and build compelling alliances that focus on achievement. Avoid hanging out with people who bring you down. Schedule a soothsaying meeting each month with fellow wizards to polish the lamp and discuss the next breathtaking venture in your plan.

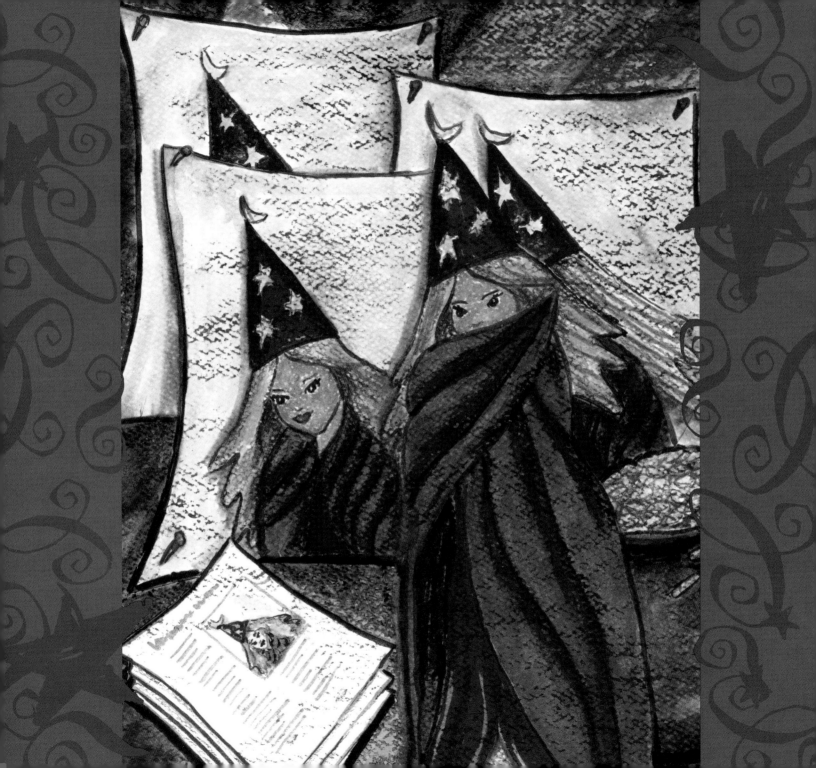

Now You See Me—
Now You See Me More

You've waved your magic wand, and now your framed CLNC® certificate hangs proudly on your wall. You're excited about being an independent business owner. Possibly you've already pulled a rabbit out of the hat and landed your first case—a friend of a friend of a friend. And you did a terrific job. But now that case is nearly finished, no others immediately in sight. What are the magic spells that make clients materialize? What is the *open sesame* to a thriving practice?

To build a business, you need sales. To generate sales, you need to market. And the real secret to marketing is another kind of magic— organized, proactive communication.

Using the following potions, you'll shed your invisibility cloak and make a magical entrance. You'll network with other wand wielders. You'll distribute business cards, brochures and information newsletters with beguiling brilliance. By integrating marketing practices into your daily routine, you'll always have an influx of cases to build a flourishing CLNC® practice. Your magician's deck of cards will hold all the tricks you need to bewitch, bedazzle and bring in the business.

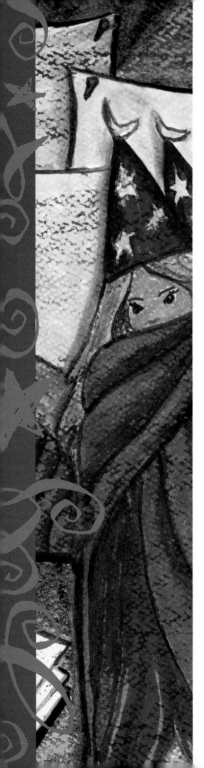

USE MAGICAL WORDS IN YOUR COMPANY NAME

Magical words are rhythmic—*abracadabra, alakazam, bibbity bobbity boo*. Notice the hard consonants, b, d, t, hard c and k? Favorite names for strong, confident fictional characters also have hard consonants such as Jack and Kate. The names Will, Lily or Cinderella, with the soft l, connote gentler, more refined characters. Choose a rhythmically captivating company name. Select with care because your name will magically define your practice.

START YOUR NAMING SPELL WITH:

✴ A list of mesmerizing names and words you like
✴ A thesaurus
✴ The *NACLNC*® Online Directory
✴ A list of non-legal nurse consultant names

OPTIONAL ELIXIR:

The local business pages

Awaken your creative mind by reading through the lists. Jot down any words or combinations that grab your attention.

Continue stirring the brew, adding similar words from your thesaurus or ideas from your friends and family.

When your brain says "enough," choose several names that stand out for you—these compile your short list.

Write one name, one word or one idea on a page, then quickly jot down every thought that surfaces. Do the same for every name on your short list.

Then read, edit and select three names that speak to you about your business.

Check the local business pages and the *NACLNC*® Online Directory to make sure your favorite name hasn't been used. Check also for similar names that might cause confusion.

Consider a name that will encompass services you provide now and into the future—don't be limiting. Or use your own name and add "Associates" in your title to provide room for growth.

Once you decide on a name, get expert advice from a CPA or attorney on whether to register under a state assumed name (DBA) or form a corporation.

MY COMPANY NAME IS

_____

JUST FOR FUN: THE MAGIC OF NUMEROLOGY

Each letter in the alphabet corresponds to a number. A=1, b=2, c=3 and so on. At i=9, the numbers start over, j=1, k=2. Assign the correct number to the letters in your company name. Then add all the numbers for a total and add the numbers in the total to reduce the sum to a single digit. ($235 = 2+3+5 = 10$, $1+0=1$). The number you arrive at has a numerological meaning. Does that number describe your business?

* *Number 1.* Unity, beginning, focused concentration, goal-striving, action, independence, originality, courage, invention, leader, self-reliant, ambition, pioneer.

* *Number 2.* Duality, division, polarity, choice, gestation, cooperation, service, harmony, support, diplomacy, patience, intuition, adaptability, partnership, receptive.

* *Number 3.* Trinity, manifestation, neutral, expression, imagination, creativity, optimism, enthusiasm, expressive, charming, humor, fun, attractive, friendly.

* *Number 4.* Practical, orderly, patient, logical, hard-working, loyal, builder, steadfast, frugal, responsible, earthy, planner, materially creative, green thumb, even tempered.

* *Number 5.* Adventure, change, freedom, exploration, variety, sensuality, unattached, curious, experienced, knowledge seeker, teacher, traveler, imagination, child-like, playful.

* *Number 6.* Harmony, beauty, nurturing, love, marriage, family, responsibility, understanding, sympathy, healing, empathic, perfectionist, order, duty, comfort, service.

* *Number 7.* Philosopher, sage, wisdom seeker, reserved, inventor, stoic, contemplative, aloof, spiritual, unusual, hidden, seeking perfection, enigma.

* *Number 8.* Achievement, abundance, executive, strength, self-disciplined, power, success, authority, psychology, entrepreneur, intensity, supervisor, provider, grandeur.

* *Number 9.* Humanitarian, compassionate, romantic, selfless, generous, philanthropic, loving, wisdom, idealist, artistic, spiritual healer, all allowing, other worldly, blending.

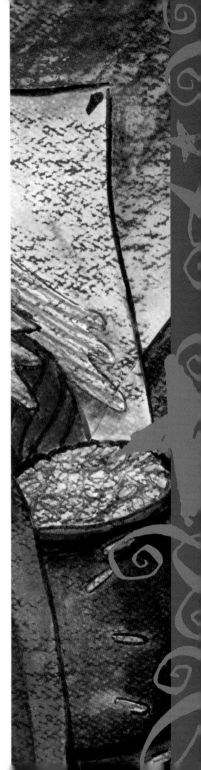

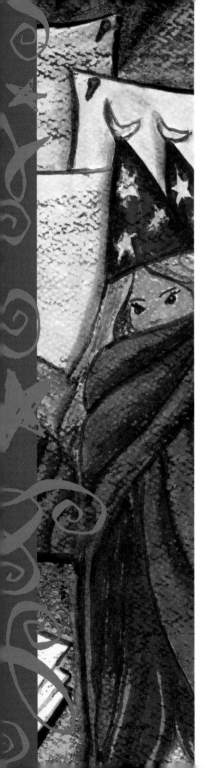

Cast Marketing Spells with Your USP

Every wizard has a specialty act, a single stunt that no other magician can do quite the same. Saw the lady in half? Read minds? Make an elephant disappear? As a Certified Legal Nurse Consultant℠, you also have unique skills, knowledge and experience that make you stand out from your peers. Use your USP (unique selling position) to brand your marketing messages and you will gain the competitive advantage.

Start your magic spell with:

✶ Your credentials and education
✶ Three of your proudest work accomplishments
✶ Any experience relevant to attorneys

Optional elixir:

The Marketing Wizard's Edge by Jay Abraham

Stir your creativity by reviewing the information above.

Create a captivating sentence defining each major accomplishment or area of experience. Refine the sentence until it presents your unique credentials and background as a benefit to attorneys. Sprinkle your assets with enough pixie dust to convince attorneys you can make them stars.

Focus your USP on your special experience and knowledge—perhaps the inner workings of hospitals, staffing issues, billing fraud or developing facility policies and procedures.

Turn a perceived disadvantage into a USP. You're over 60? No problem, age equals experience. Under 25? Youth has the advantage of cutting-edge viewpoints.

Highlight your USP in your promotional package, interviews and every time you meet anyone. Use it to position yourself uniquely. Practice your USP until it rolls off your tongue naturally and easily. If you sound like you're selling, it may be too formal.

My USP is _____

> **Shaman's Secret:** Services don't sell at $150 an hour, expertise sells. This is the time to mesmerize, dazzle and charm, to use your sleight-of-hand and turn all your nursing and CLNC® assets into attorney-client benefits. You've got the magic. Now is the time to flaunt it.

Examples of dazzling USPs

Clinical: "I have ten years clinical experience in critical care and have analyzed medical and nursing care daily for ten years." *The benefit to the attorney?* "I can review any critical care or med-surg issue quickly and easily."

Management: "I have eight years experience in nursing management. In addition to being an expert on clinical standards of care, I'm also an expert on staffing, delegation and accreditation issues."

Dazzle Prospects with Your Promotional Package

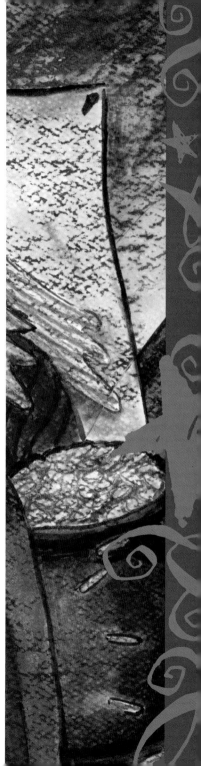

When old-time wizards came to town, they rode in wagons painted with brightly colored drawings depicting the highlights of their act. The drawings dazzled, intrigued and enticed the townsfolk to line up and buy their tickets. Your promotional package is your wizard's wagon. It dazzles, intrigues and entices attorneys to purchase your CLNC® services.

Conjure Your Unique Brand With:

- ✴ Business cards
- ✴ Resume
- ✴ Letter of introduction
- ✴ Marketing brochure
- ✴ Risk-free guarantee
- ✴ Sample work product
- ✴ Letters of recommendation
- ✴ Information newsletter
- ✴ Articles related to legal nurse consulting
- ✴ CLNC® Marketing LaunchBox

Optional Elixir:

A writer and designer for best impact

Mail only five or ten promotional packages each week. Then follow up seven days later with a phone call. Make sure your risk-free guarantee is clearly visible in your promotional package.

Take your resume and sample work product to all interviews.

Send your information newsletter to every attorney-client and prospect. Collect relevant articles on recent medical issues that might affect their cases and mail monthly.

Consider including a pen or small note pad imprinted with your company name inside each promotional package. The added bulk entices the prospect to open the envelope. The enclosure will stay around long after you or your promo package, guaranteeing that you won't be doing a disappearing act any time soon.

Keep prospects on your mailing list for at least a year. Keep clients on your mailing list forever.

> **Wizard's Tip:** Don't expect to get a response after only one mailing. Marketing, like conjuring, becomes more successful with repetition. After your follow-up phone call, mail again and again. Be patient, persistent, charming and enthusiastic, and you won't have to kiss a frog to turn prospects into clients.

The CLNC® Marketing LaunchBox Magically Conjures Up Business

Professionally designed brochures, business cards and letterhead stationery designed by Vickie Milazzo Institute are instantly ready for you to start marketing to attorneys.

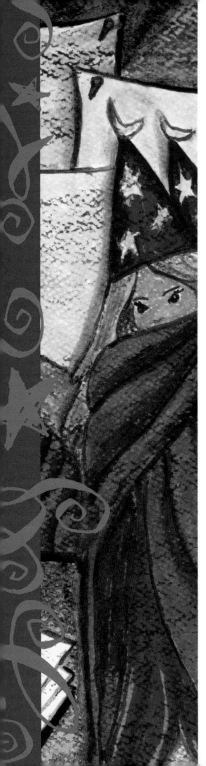

Never Leave Home Without Your Most Portable Potion

The easiest potion you'll ever make is also one of the most powerful. It's the marketing tool you carry everywhere. It's the *open sesame* rune you will cast into the pocket of every attorney, every prospect, every person you meet. It's a small, portable and mighty potion that will spread your name throughout the kingdom as surely as a thousand owls.

Start your magic potion with:

✴ Your name and credentials
✴ Your title
✴ Your company name
✴ Addresses—mail and delivery
✴ Phone number
✴ Fax number
✴ Email and website addresses
✴ Your CLNC® T-shirt or polo
✴ CLNC® Marketing LaunchBox business card

Embellish your creation with a fascinating logo, wizard's mark or other graphic. Use irresistible color. A creative and memorable business card (like the cards in the CLNC® Marketing LaunchBox) will make a lasting impression and remain in a prospect's file long after plain cards have been forgotten.

Make your card a keeper by including a bewitching ingredient on the back that attorneys will want to retain—a calendar, your CLNC® services, your areas of nursing expertise, a magic incantation or a list of medical abbreviations.

Carry your business card up your sleeve and magically make one appear every time you meet a friend, attorney, another wizard—or anybody and everybody who comes within three feet of you. Wear your CLNC® shirt to every casual event. Mail a business card with your letter of introduction, brochure and letters of recommendation to all prospects.

> **Enchanter's Tip:** At the same time you print your business card, print postcards using the same irresistible colors and artwork. Make the postcard a size that can be mailed as is or slipped into an envelope. You will find hundreds of uses—a quick thank you, a reminder, an attachment to a report—and the total cost will be less than if you printed the cards separately.

*Always carry your cards
in a business card case to keep them
dazzlingly crisp and impressive.*

Write Your Resume to Live Your Fairy Tale

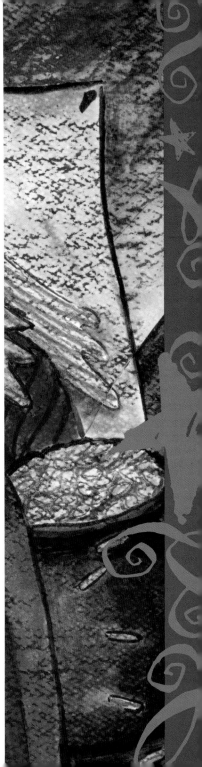

To be successful, your resume must reflect the difference between an elementary bag of tricks and the advanced technique of a master wizard. The keen conjurer understands that a platform of reality and truth are the underpinnings of the best sleight-of-hand illusion. In a resume, you want to dazzle attorneys with your brilliance, not with hoax. And *abracadabra* all the wonders of this practical magic are already in your illusionist's toolbox.

Assemble your illusionist's tools:

* Your unique selling position (USP)
* Your qualifications and expertise
* Your education
* Your CLNC® certification
* Results of any pertinent research
* Reports or articles you've published
* Professional conferences you've attended

Consider your audience—attorneys who need your magical services to help them win cases. Review the materials above and highlight specific information pertinent to potential attorney-clients.

Organize your ideas. Then summarize your strengths in an overview paragraph with five bullet points that reflect the benefits you can provide.

Highlight your nursing expertise that no other healthcare provider possesses, such as quality assurance, policy and procedure development, case management or risk management.

List legal nurse consulting work before your other work experience.

Be 100% honest, but education degrees and certification dates can do a disappearing act.

Take a break to get a fresh look at what you've written, then edit. Cut the fluff.

Print on professional letterhead (included in the CLNC® Marketing LaunchBox).

> **Conjurer's Tip:** A resume for a consulting expert should be one page, tight, punchy and to the point. Like the one that should appear in the *NACLNC*® Online Directory. The curriculum vitae (CV) for a testifying expert should be as long as necessary to include everything you've ever done, detailed to show you're the expert. Bewitch, bedazzle, beguile your audience and be specific.

A resume checklist

* Name, title, credentials, address, phone, fax, email address, website URL.
* 1st section—Summary of qualifications. Include five statements identifying your USP. Illustrate your unique qualifications to work as a Certified Legal Nurse Consultant[CM].
* 2nd section—Professional experience, starting with the most recent.
* 3rd section—Education, certifications.
* 4th section—Publications and presentations.

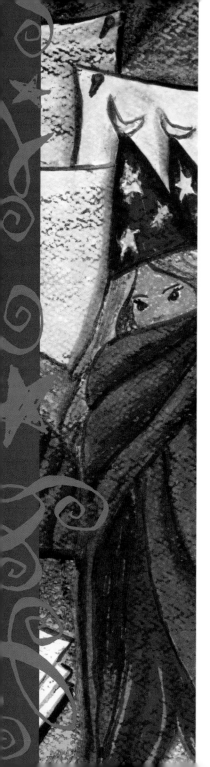

Fly with Brochures— They're Swifter Than Broomsticks

Even with a lightning fast broomstick, you can only call on so many attorney-prospects in a day, but a handful of brochures can deliver your message to hundreds of potential clients. While it will not take the place of face-to-face marketing, a fabulous brochure can magically open the door for an interview. Use this spell to create an attention-getting, informative door-opener that will bewitch prospects into contracting your services.

Start your magic spell with:

* Your unique selling position (USP)
* Your qualifications and experience
* A budget, even a humble one—and the money to implement it
* Creativity, enthusiasm and your wizard's thinking cap
* CLNC® Marketing LaunchBox brochure

Optional elixir:

A writer and/or graphic designer

Begin with a benefit to the reader. Use catchy, easy-to-grasp, captivating headlines, especially on the cover. Be specific about your offer. State what you can do and how your service will help attorneys win cases. Write your brochure copy using the six Cs:

1. **Clear.** Use language your prospect won't have to puzzle over. Avoid medical terms and wizard's words that an average reader might not understand. Use short sentences and action-oriented verbs such as *developed,* *created, supervised, managed*. Be specific about your accomplishments.

2. **Concise.** Eliminate unnecessary words, inflated phrases and repetitions. A good brochure should tell just enough to interest the reader and entice response.

3. **Consistent.** Use the same tone and style throughout. Check the use of your magician's logo and company name for consistency.

4. **Credible.** Use positive, upbeat statements. Express your expertise and experience in glowing terms, but avoid sounding as if you're exaggerating the facts. Be believable. Boldly state your risk-free guarantee.

5. **Current.** Check for correct address, phone, fax and email information, prominently positioned. Make sure all CLNC® services and sorceries are included.

6. **Correct.** Proofread your brochure three times, and have at least one other person who is not involved in the process read it for clarity.

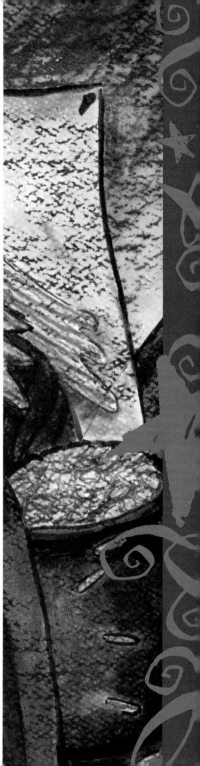

Soothsayer's Advice: About 50% of your readers are *information oriented* and will eagerly read every word. The other 50% are *action oriented* and only want the highlights. To captivate 100% of your prospects, break up your brochure copy with enchanting white space and with subheadings that provide an overview. Information-oriented readers will be mesmerized by the details, while action-oriented readers can quickly scan the fascinating subheadings.

Tell the reader exactly when and how to respond. While it might seem obvious to you, research shows that your marketing pieces must be specific in stating what the reader should do to receive the benefits offered. Example: *Call now to schedule a free consultation.*

5-STEP BROCHURE

1. Get the attorney's attention with benefit-focused headlines.

2. Elaborate briefly on your offer and on the CLNC® magic you can perform.

3. Briefly state your experience and why the reader should believe you.

4. Restate the benefit, along with your risk-free guarantee, and give examples of specific types of cases on which you've worked.

5. Include a call to action, telling the reader what to do next to receive the benefit.

90-SECOND TEST

Ask someone who is not familiar with your services to review your brochure for 90 seconds and then identify:

✓ Your target reader
✓ What you are offering

Make sure the response is exactly what you intended before heading for the printer. Or go with the already-proven brochures that appear in the CLNC® Marketing LaunchBox.

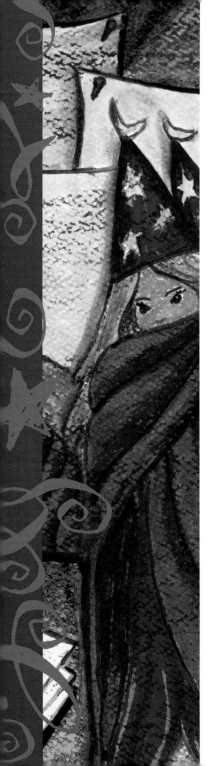

Showcase Your Samples with Beguiling Brilliance

Eel's eyes, toad's toes, unicorn horn—and *bibbity, bobbity, boo!* The sorcerer mixes her elixirs and lines them up enticingly on a shelf in sparkling bottles. She is showcasing her wares. You, too, must showcase your work product to dazzle attorneys with your brilliance.

Assemble your conjurer's tools:

* A brief report
* A single page of a chronological timeline
* Several pages of a comprehensive report documenting adherences to and deviations from the standards of care
* A sample search of the scientific literature
* A dictionary
* A thesaurus

Optional elixirs:

Core Curriculum for Legal Nurse Consulting® textbook

Advanced CLNC® Toolkit

Create your sample work product as carefully as the finest elixir. Make it sparkle.

Use language an average reader will easily understand. No abbreviations or medical jargon.

Read the sample three times for grammatical and typographical errors.

Ask a knowledgeable friend to proofread the final product for clarity.

Bind the sample in a professional-looking folder.

Create a variety of samples to match the attorney you are marketing to.

Showcase your samples on your website.

> **Sorcerer's Tip:** Your sample work product is a wonder-working marketing tool that makes an irresistible impact on attorneys. It shows that you can communicate clearly. You not only can do the research and recognize deviations from the recognized standards of care, you can also create a high-quality report that helps your attorney-client make the case. Your brilliance shines and weaves its beguiling spell.

USE A SLEIGHT-OF-HAND PLAN AND YOUR MARKET APPEARS

"Abracadabra," says the magician, waving his wand over the hat. Instantly, out pops a rabbit. Could it be so easy? With the right strategy, yes. A master magician plans each sleight-of-hand trick long before taking the stage. As a CLNC® business owner, you must devise your own artful trickery for tapping into your market. Then, *abracadabra!* Your market appears.

ASSEMBLE YOUR MAGIC POTIONS:

* A contact and prospect list
* A promo package: business cards, cover letter, brochure, sample report, post cards
* A tracking system for follow-up
* A news release announcing your new CLNC® practice
* A dress-for-success power suit
* A dash of confidence
* Your unique selling position (USP)
* CLNC® pillars of marketing

CAST THE RUNES TO FORETELL YOUR FUTURE:

Successful marketing begins with a plan. What are your strengths? Are you outgoing and people-oriented? Then use that magical charisma. Are you a task-focused analyst? Then conjure some devilishly clever tactics.

Send out your news release.

Mark your calendar with selected networking events and attorney seminars and conferences you will attend.

Block out your most energized hours each day for follow-up calls and cold-calling your prospect list.

Schedule interviews.

Don your sorcerer's power suit and dazzle your prospect with your knowledge, expertise and USP.

Ask for the sale.

Clairvoyant's Prophesy: The most successful marketing plans are simple and specific. Spend 20 minutes forecasting your month, ten minutes planning your week, five minutes scheduling your day, then open your heart and mind to whatever appears. You'll pull success out of your hat with the ease of a master trickster.

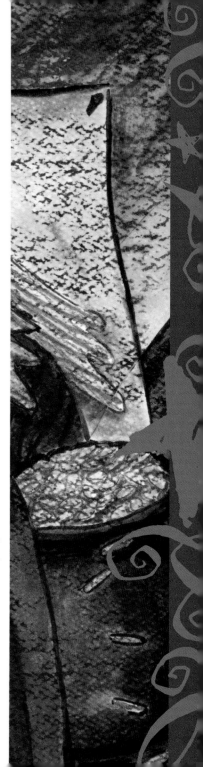

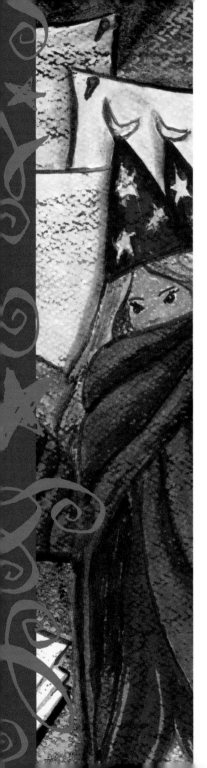

BEWITCH PROSPECTS WITH YOUR MAGICAL ENTRANCE

Making a good first impression is a crucial advantage for every wizard, and it does not require spinning around in the air on your Nimbus 2000 broomstick. In networking situations and all business interactions making a bewitching impression means looking into your crystal ball to know what to do and when to do it.

Start your enchanting spell with:

* A cup of confidence
* A pound of enthusiasm
* A heaping measure of consideration
* An ounce of foresight

Optional elixir:

Emily Post's The Etiquette Advantage in Business by **Peggy Post and Peter Post**

Approach all networking and business interactions as opportunities to showcase your CLNC® magic and open doors to sales opportunities. Always respect the time and opinions of others and help them as much or more than you are helped. The smart CLNC® sorcerer establishes rapport long before conjuring a favor or even presenting a business card.

Arrive early with your plan for making the people you meet feel good about themselves. Carry yourself with confidence and smile. Look lively and genuinely glad to be there.

Focus your attention off yourself and onto others. Keep the conversation flowing. Plan to make the people you meet feel good about themselves. Ask polite and captivating questions about the family, friends and social interests of others. Really listen to the answers. The most scintillating conversationalist is not the one who is always talking but the one who cares enough to listen.

Learn the art of making enchanting introductions:

* To appear respectful, professional and powerful, stand for all introductions. Make eye contact, smile and give a firm handshake.

* At a business luncheon or dinner, introduce yourself to the people seated on both sides of you.

* While social introductions are based on age and gender, business introductions are based on hierarchy. Start with the person of highest position; say that name first, then make the

introduction. An exception is when introducing a client—always say the client's name first. "Mr. Attorney, this is Joe Smith, president of Money Bank."

- When introducing a woman, use Ms. unless informed otherwise.
- An elected official takes precedence. Always use honorifics and titles.

Wizard's Tip: Include a conversation starter in your introductions. When introducing yourself, include a humorous, surprising or definitive comment about what you do. If you know of an interest you share with that person—golf, boating, travel, crystal gazing, broomstick aerobics— mention that as well. When introducing two people to each other, provide more than just names. Give specific mutual business or hobby interests to break the ice. You'll discover these charming tidbits by careful listening, and you'll magically establish connections to ease those first awkward moments. For that simple courtesy, you'll shine as the brightest star in the room.

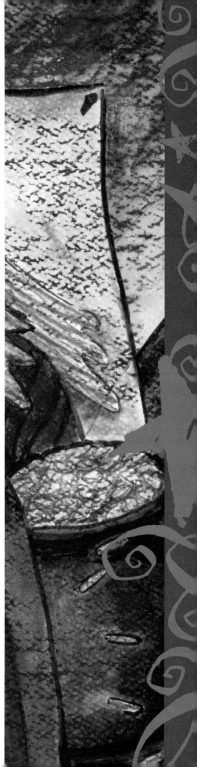

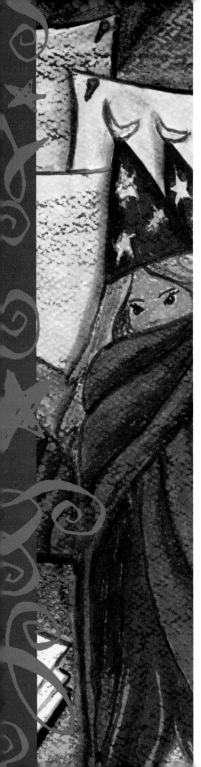

Network with Other Wand Wielders

Your next-door neighbor might be an attorney who desperately needs the services of a Certified Legal Nurse Consultant^{CM}. Your elevator companion could be the office manager for the city's largest legal firm. Your dentist's spouse could be the lawyer who just landed that big medical case you read about. Anyone you meet could be the Merlin who waves the wand and opens your market. It doesn't take telepathy to find out who is standing next to you. All you need to do is *ask*.

Prepare your bag of tricks:

* Business cards in a bewitchingly attractive case
* Your most enchanting smile
* A captivating ten-word explanation of what you do
* Promotional packets for follow-up
* A contact list of everyone you know
* Your CLNC® T-shirt or polo shirt
* A commitment to systemize networking

Conjure a roomful of contacts:

Attend events. Networking luncheons, church events, birthday parties, little league games—any gathering offers an opportunity to ask the magic question: *Who do you know who practices law or interfaces with attorneys?* Practically everyone you meet will know at least one attorney and important contact.

Contact everyone you know to ferret out more wand wielders and add more events to your calendar. Ask everyone the magic question.

Even create your own events, such as tea time or lunch out.

Stir yourself into the gathering. Go with an objective to meet at least three people and to walk away with at least three names of attorneys you can call. Leave your shyness at home.

Arrive early and station yourself near the door to meet people as they come in.

Or hang out near the food and laugh about how quickly the food is magically disappearing.

Ask people about themselves and listen. Then give your ten-word introduction and ask the magic question: *Who do you know who practices law or interfaces with attorneys?*

Follow up with everyone you meet by emailing or dropping a thank-you card.

My next networking event will be

_____

_____

_____

_____

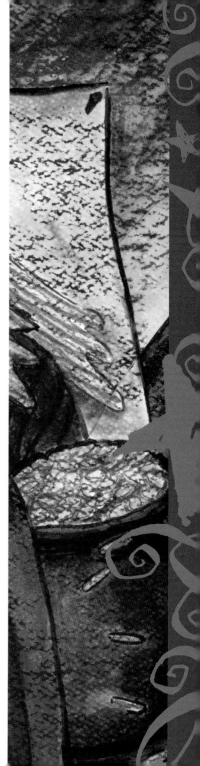

> **Soothsayer's Advice:** Remember the three-foot rule. Always be prepared with your business card up your sleeve. You never know where or when, but you'll bump into attorneys at the most unexpected places. You'll need to pull a card out quickly. Talk to everyone you see—in the grocery check-out line, at your kids' soccer game. Wear your CLNC® shirt in every casual situation, and be ready to give your ten-word introduction to anyone who comes within three feet of you. Forget Merlin, you have your own magic wand.

Favorite examples of unexpected networking locations that paid off big

- Standing in line at Starbucks, an attorney noticed the T-shirt slogan and asked, "What's a CLNC® consultant?"

- On a hiking trail, strangers started up a conversation. One was an attorney, the other a Certified Legal Nurse Consultant^{CM}.

- At a football game, an attorney was sitting next to a CLNC® consultant. She received her first case from him the next day.

- In a bank, a CLNC® consultant asked, "Do attorneys ever come in here?" The banker pointed out an attorney sitting in the lobby. That attorney was her first client.

- In an elevator, a CLNC® consultant struck up a conversation and stepped out with a client.

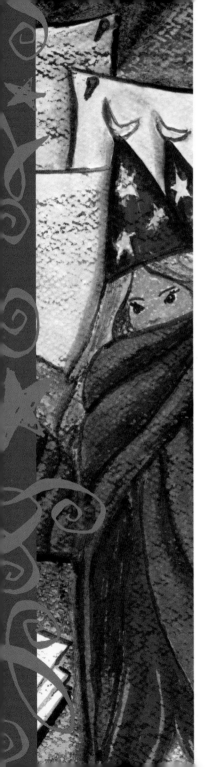

 # BVILD A GOLDEN PROSPECT LIST

Attorneys need your CLNC® services. And for the growth of your business, a targeted list of attorney-prospects is more powerful than any lucky charm. It's the yellow brick road to a flourishing practice. With one name and a touch of your sorcerer's skill, you can start your prospect list. Quicker than *shazaam*, it will become a bottomless resource for new business.

ASSEMBLE YOUR ALCHEMIST'S TOOLS:

* Local and national attorney directories, such as *Martindale-Hubbell*
* Names gathered at social and professional networking organizations
* Legal reporters, journals and other publications, such as *Lawyers USA*
* The Internet
* The Yellow Pages

OPTIONAL ELIXIR:

Attend or exhibit at a legal seminar or conference and use the attendee/exhibitor list.

Condense your resource pool by location, starting with attorneys in your area and branching out from there.

Confirm the accuracy of your list by researching the attorney's website and locating the firm in *Martindale-Hubbell*. Gather as much information as possible to personalize the marketing to his practice and needs. Start from the middle of a directory, rather than the beginning. You can bet the As, Bs and Cs receive more calls than others.

Qualify your prospects by the quality of the lead, with direct referrals being the most desirable.

Transfer your list to a contact management software such as ACT!® or a prospect grid. Across the top, ascribe such headings as Referral Source, Date of First Contact, Follow-up Phone Call Made, Follow-up Brochure Sent and Interview Date. List the names and contact information down the side of the grid, then record each communication and continue to qualify each prospect according to the response you receive.

Enchanter's Secret: Your prospect list, like a road paved with gold, needs occasional polishing. Add at least one new name per week. Ask everyone you know and meet. Note the resources that result in the best prospects. Keep your list current. And keep in touch. A lawyer who does not need your CLNC® services today might land a case tomorrow requiring precisely the magic you can deliver.

SHED YOUR INVISIBILITY CLOAK

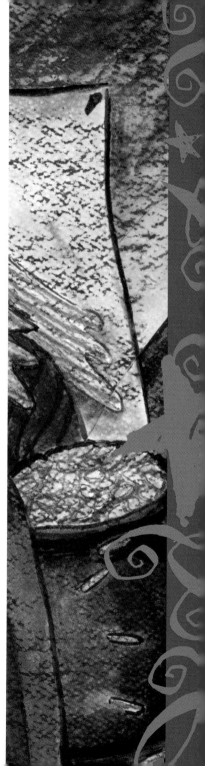

A nurse's uniform is like an invisibility cloak. While you stand out from ordinary people, you blend in, even vanish among your peers. As a CLNC® consultant you want to shed your invisibility cloak to stand out among other Certified Legal Nurse Consultants℠. Shedding the scrubs is only the beginning. Every good magician has a top hat, a magic wand and a special deck of cards. Use this spell to create the magic tools that will banish invisibility.

Start your visibility spell with:

★ Your unique selling position (USP)

★ Your personal style—clothing, manner, presence

★ Your bedazzling background

★ Your integrity, expertise and responsiveness

★ Your intriguing interests and hobbies

Stand on the cutting edge. Educate yourself continually about your profession. Attend the *NACLNC*® Conference every year.

Break away from the competition by experimenting with new skills and potions. Dare to expand the borders of your comfort zone. Be the first in your magic kingdom to provide a new CLNC® service.

Stay one step ahead and set the standard.

Personalize your professional relationships. Identify common interests such as the church you attend, hobbies you enjoy, family similarities and restaurants you frequent. Look for common bonds such as favorite vacation spots, school ties or ancestral heritage. Use anything you find in common with an attorney-prospect or client to distinguish yourself.

Never take attorneys for granted. Do an outstanding job each time, every time. Treat every case as if it is your most important case.

> **Sorcerer's Secret:** A wizard is only as popular as his latest, most spellbinding spectacle. Let competition bring out the best in you. Setting yourself apart from your competitors pushes you to a higher level while it builds your confidence and self-esteem. Don't obsess over competition, but allow your competition to propel you to excellence.

A checklist for visibility

- A bold brand.
- Regular face-to-face communication with attorney-prospects and clients.
- Information newsletter.
- Speaking engagements at legal conferences.
- A spellbinding website.
- Plenty of networking engagements.
- Strong letters of recommendation.
- Articles published in legal journals.
- Attendance at the *NACLNC*® Conference.

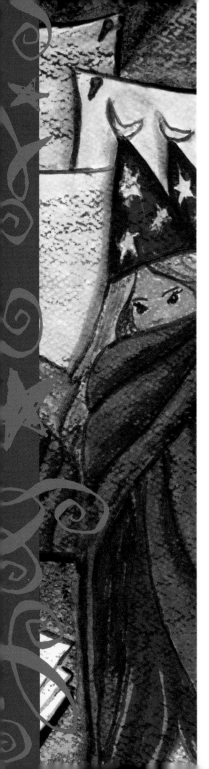

Bedazzle Attorneys with Information Newsletters

The Pied Piper played a few bewitching notes and enticed all the children of Hamlin to follow him. Similarly, a few bewitching words can work an entrancement with attorneys. Attorneys need your knowledge, talent and skill. The magic flute that will attract them is your information newsletter.

Assemble your magician's tools:

* A list of prospects and clients
* Ten topics you can easily write about
* A schedule—monthly, bimonthly, quarterly
* A budget

Optional elixir:

A writer and graphic designer

Envision your information newsletter arriving on the attorney's desk. Is it electronic or traditional print? The headlines on the front page grab attention—what are those headlines? What makes your target prospect read your newsletter?

Forecast the next six issues. Include a major topic and a few minor topics such as new standards and healthcare regulations, managed care issues or your involvement in an interesting medical case.

Keep the newsletter educational and informational. Leave overt sales to your brochure or ad copy. Include a short bio, your photo, name, company name, contact information and your risk-free guarantee. Each month, highlight the benefits of one valuable CLNC® service.

Turn boring topics into exciting headlines. Use such key words or phrases as *New...*, *Finally...*, *At Last...*, *How to...*, *4 Easy Steps to...*, *5 Ways to Conquer...*

Weave in, when possible, the story of how you made a positive difference in the outcome of a case.

> **Wizard's Tip:** With every issue, your newsletter bedazzles attorneys with your credibility and reminds them you're there, available and ready to help them mesmerize the jury on their next case. Whistle a few bewitching notes while you conjure the words that will captivate, entrance and entice prospects to use your services.

How valuable is a newsletter?

Consider the potential yearly income from a single attorney who elects to use your CLNC® services after receiving your newsletter. It could easily be $10,000, $20,000 or even $40,000. Now consider the cost to produce and mail the newsletter for a year—$500 to $1,000 plus a bit of your time. You'll discover an information newsletter is a highly effective marketing tool at a nominal cost.

TURN LEAD INTO GOLD BY EXHIBITING

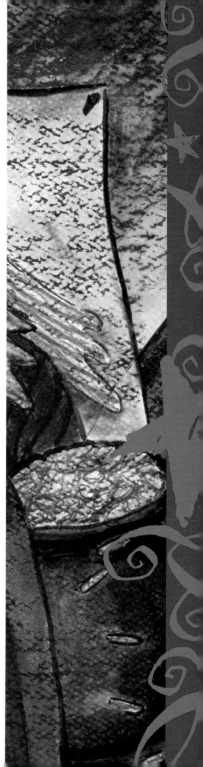

A mid lightning flashes, smoke and swirls of pixie dust a wizard materializes. It's show time! An audience gathers to *ooh* and *aah*. The magician performs her sleight-of-hand, and the audience leaves impressed. For any CLNC® sorcerer, exhibiting at legal conferences is your opportunity to perform your own lightshow.

FOR YOUR MESMERIZING PERFORMANCE, ASSEMBLE:

* A table with an attractive cover—usually supplied by the conference
* A simple stand-up display board—available at office, art supply or hobby stores
* Samples pages of your work product
* A list of attorney benefits
* Pictures and photos if applicable
* An eye catcher—anatomical skeleton or heart
* Your promotional package
* Name and address forms for attorneys without business cards
* A bowl or magician's hat to collect names
* A prize to give away, e.g., first screening free
* Enthusiasm, courage, patience and persistence
* Comfortable and attractive shoes

Arrive early to set up. Use color, graphics, fresh flowers, music—whatever will attract favorable attention for you and your magic show. Allow enough time to freshen up after you put the finishing sparkle on your display.

Stand in front of, not behind, the table. Initiate communication with a smile, a few words and a handshake. Savor your 30-second introduction on the tip of your tongue. Show your enthusiastic interest in everyone you meet.

Attend the conference networking functions and introduce yourself to attorneys.

Visit other exhibitors' tables, exchange cards and ask them to introduce you to their favorite attorneys. Mix, mingle and meet—this is the purpose of your exhibit.

Follow up promptly on every lead.

MY NEXT EXHIBIT OPPORTUNITY IS

> **Shaman's Secret:** Exhibiting at attorney conferences is a captivating way to network with attorney-prospects. Razzle-dazzle, lightning flashes, clouds of pixie dust and leads, leads, leads. Some legal nurse consultants consider exhibiting to be costly. Focus on conferences that will net high results, and you could be the only CLNC® consultant with your own magical lightshow.

A SAMPLE SPELL THAT WORKS MAGIC

When your audience dwindles, attend the conference sessions. Sit beside an attorney and make friends. Exchange cards with at least one attorney at each session every day of the conference.

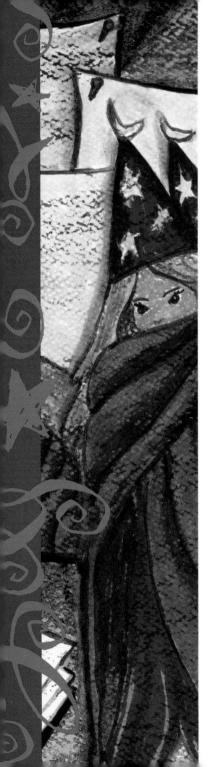

Advertise to Spin Your Magic Show Starward

You are there—even when you're not. The magic of advertising enables you to be two, three, even a thousand places at once showing prospects why they need your CLNC® services. At the same time, you are working magic at your office or traveling to consult other wizards. Don your sorcerer's cloak and pointy hat, nibble a few cauldron cakes or licorice wands while you conjure a spectacular advertising program.

Start your magic spell with:

* Your unique selling position (USP)
* Your qualifications and experience
* A benefits-focused headline
* A budget and the money to implement it
* A list of legal publications
* Creativity, patience and persistence
* *NACLNC*® Online Directory
* Vickie Milazzo Institute's trial-attorney ad

Optional elixir:

A writer and/or graphic designer

Start by brainstorming your goals. Decide what specific sorcery you want the ads to do for you. Brand your name on the audience? Pave the way for cold calls? Entice an attorney-prospect to call you? Encourage drop-ins at an exhibit? Answers to these questions may seem obvious, and you might be inclined to say "All of the above." That would generally be a mistake. A specific objective attains better results than a cluttered approach. While you may reap benefits in several areas, start with a single concrete goal in mind.

Keep it simple. Write a clear, concise message that states the benefits of using your services and the action needed to receive that benefit.

Research the publications you want to use and determine the cost of advertising at least three consecutive months. Calculate this cost in your overall budget.

Stretch your advertising dollar. A small, creative ad repeated often is better than a large ad you can afford to run only once or twice. Repetition reaps rewards.

Save money by addng your name, specialty and phone number to Vickie Milazzo Institute's full-page ad in one of the leading national publications for trial attorneys.

Add Premium Features to your *NACLNC*® Online Directory listing so that attorneys see you first.

Track your effectiveness. Ask new attorney-clients how they learned about you.

> **Soothsayer's Tip:** Once you decide to advertise, make a commitment to a continued campaign. The more times you run an ad, the lower your cost per ad. The more the ad is seen, the more it will razzle-dazzle and enchant, and the more it becomes credible in the eyes of your audience. Remember: one lifetime client could pay for your advertising ten times over.

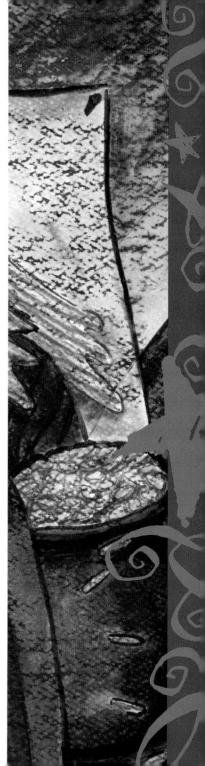

4 steps to a compelling ad

✓ Get attention with a benefit to the reader.
✓ Briefly elaborate why this benefit is important at this time.
✓ Briefly state your credentials and why the reader should believe you.
✓ Call for action—tell the reader exactly what to do to get the benefit.

Sample ad:

CLNC® Review Wins Cases

Discover hidden medical facts that will give you the winning edge in your next case. As a Certified Legal Nurse Consultant℠, I can quickly review medical records for relevant facts and standards. Call now for more information: (your company name and phone number).

How often should you advertise? The answer may surprise you.

What are people actually thinking as they read your ad? Thomas Smith, a London businessman, offered this insight to advertisers in 1885. It is still applicable today.

1. The first time people look at any given ad, they don't even see it.
2. The second time, they don't notice it.
3. The third time, they are aware that it is there.
4. The fourth time, they have a fleeting sense that they've seen it somewhere before.
5. The fifth time, they actually read the ad.
6. The sixth time, they thumb their nose at it.
7. The seventh time, they start to get a little irritated with it.
8. The eighth time, they start to think, "Here's that confounded ad again."
9. The ninth time, they start to wonder if they may be missing out on something.
10. The tenth time, they ask their friends and neighbors if they've tried it.
11. The eleventh time, they wonder how the company is paying for all these ads.
12. The twelfth time, they start to think that it must be a good product.
13. The thirteenth time, they start to feel the product has value.
14. The fourteenth time, they start to remember wanting a product exactly like this for a long time.
15. The fifteenth time, they start to yearn for it because they can't afford to buy it.
16. The sixteenth time, they accept the fact that they will buy it sometime in the future.
17. The seventeenth time, they make a note to buy the product.
18. The eighteenth time, they curse their poverty for not allowing them to buy this terrific product.
19. The nineteenth time, they count their money very carefully.
20. The twentieth time prospects see the ad, they buy what is offered.

In other words, if your ad campaigns aren't showing a return after six weeks, don't give up hope!

From the *Sales and Marketing Report*, 800.878.5331, ragan.com. Used with permission.

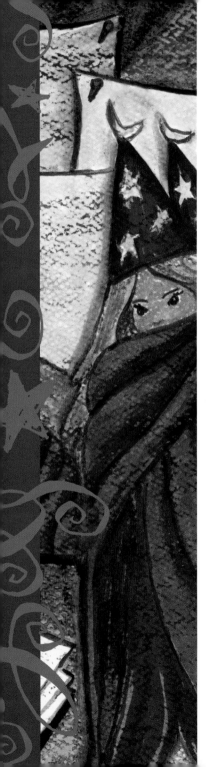

GO BEYOND SMOKE AND MIRRORS WITH PUBLIC RELATIONS

Within hours after Snow White went to live with seven dwarves at a cottage in the woods, the wicked queen knew her whereabouts. Was the queen's talking mirror really magic? Or did the buzz come from pixies, elves, squirrels and other woodland creatures? Public relations is the ultimate word-of-mouth advertising, a magic potion—not only for wicked queens but for any smart wizard's recognition and credibility. Use the following spell to start the buzz about your business.

START YOUR MAGIC SPELL WITH:

* Announcement cards for any event
* A 20-minute talk on a topic attorneys want to know about
* An article on the same topic
* A list of business and legal organizations that need speakers
* A list of periodicals that reach attorneys
* A brief marketing survey
* A website
* An information newsletter
* A news release on your newsworthy event

Publicize the opening of your new CLNC® business, your next speaking engagement, where you will be exhibiting, a presentation or your participation in and the satisfactory outcome of a high-profile case. Send out announcement cards or an information newsletter to clients, prospects, pixies, elves, fellow wizards and anyone who might have an interest.

Tap into a larger audience by writing a news release and sending it to local newspapers, newsletters and online magazines.

Speak at business associations and legal conferences. Speaking is a powerful vehicle for positive public relations. Send a notice of the event to local calendars—newspapers, radio and TV. Some local TV stations provide calendars for their audience. Repurpose your talk into an article for your information newsletter or other publications aimed at attorneys. Don't forget electronic versions of these periodicals.

Participate in charitable functions. Often your name and company will be listed in the advertising materials.

Align with your CLNC® peers. For additional exposure, attend the *NACLNC®* Conference every year.

Conduct a one-hour presentation for a law firm about new standards in healthcare.

Create a marketing survey which includes questions about legal nurse consulting. Mail the survey to clients and prospects, and use it as a handout at speaking events and conference exhibits.

MARKETING SURVEY

Create a simple marketing survey for your prospects or previous clients. Not only will you gain important information, you will stimulate interest for your services as a Certified Legal Nurse Consultant[CM]. Here are some tips for creating the survey. The response you get might surprise you.

- Make the survey short—approximately five to six questions.
- Make your questions easy to answer with yes/no or multiple choice responses.
- Leave room for respondents to write additional comments.

- Include a postage-paid business reply envelope or double postcard if sent by mail.
- Provide a place for permission to send marketing materials.
- Make it easy for prospects to sign up for your free information newsletter.

Wizard's Wisdom: Public relations is a magical window through which the public views your company. Think of everything you do as an opportunity to enchant and mesmerize.

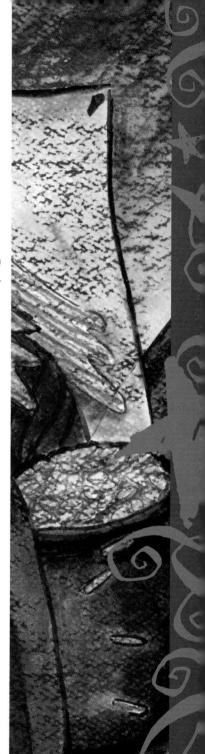

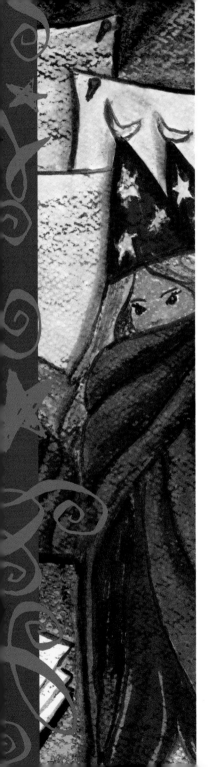

 # HERALD THE NEWS

Like a scroll that announces the king's ball or a fanfare of trumpets that precedes a momentous pronouncement, your good news needs a carrier to spread it throughout your kingdom. That artful carrier is called a "news release." Use the following incantation to brew up fame.

Start your magic spell with:

* A newsworthy event
* A list of local TV and radio stations, newspapers and other publications
* Up-to-the-minute contact information for each listing
* A stack of newspapers and legal magazines

Optional elixir:

The website PublicityHound.com

Create your one-page news release, double-spaced, with one-inch margins. Write the announcement in pyramid style, with the most important information at the top and the least important at the bottom. The publication editor will cut text from the bottom up to fit the space allotted. For ideas on how to write the text, check out articles in your newspaper.

Be sure the information in your release is newsworthy. Avoid words and phrases that sound too salesy such as *incredible* or *breakthrough*.

Triple-check all of your information for accuracy, especially names, phone numbers and addresses. A good trick is to read it several ways, even out loud and backwards. Have someone else proof your release.

Call each media organization to which you plan to send your news releases and request a media kit and submission requirements. Get the name of the wizard who accepts material for the business or medical section.

Add your contact information to the top left corner of the news release.

Fax, email or mail the news release to the appropriate contact as well as to the editor.

Follow up in a polite manner to be sure your news release was received. Being perceived as a devilish pest is a sure way *not* to get your material published.

Actively scour newspapers and legal publications for opportunities to write timely Letters to the Editor. This is the easiest way of all to get published.

> **Herald's Tip:** After writing your release, capture those well thought-out words and make them work for you in other magical ways. Sprinkle some of the more dazzling phrases in your promotional package or information newsletter. Having your news release published could bring distinction and esteem to your CLNC® business. Get permission to make copies and send the news that you *are* news to your prospects and attorney-clients. Include professionally created copies of the clipping in your promotional package.

Examples of newsworthy topics

* Achieving CLNC® status
* Nurse Charting a New Career and Making a Difference
* Why Consumers Should Have a CLNC® Consultant on Their Litigation Team

KEEP CLIENTS REAPPEARING

You'll spend 80% more time and energy attracting new attorney-clients than you will in retaining the clients you have. And that 80% marketing time is non-billable. Is there a CLNC® service one satisfied lawyer uses that other attorneys don't yet know about? Do you have expertise you haven't even placed on the table? The secret formula for client retention goes deeper than merely doing a good job. And this magic potion will cast a spell to bring your attorney-clients back again and again.

CREATE YOUR POTION WITH THE 3 RS:

1. **Respect.** Collaboratively assess what's needed, then do what you say you will do with integrity, quality and commitment to the case. Make each attorney feel as if she is your only client.

2. **Response.** Anticipate the attorney-client's needs. Meet or beat their deadlines and always provide quality work product. Give the wizard's lagniappe of a little more value than expected.

3. **Repetition.** Anticipate the client's future needs, send a follow-up letter and follow up again on a regular basis. Ask for feedback: "What features of this work product were especially helpful? Is there anything I could eliminate next time to save you time and money?" Make sure your next work product reflects that you heard their feedback. Send a sample of a CLNC® service the client hasn't yet used, such as developing deposition questions. And be sure to ask for the next case.

Mix your opportunities for repeat business with good communication, accessibility and enthusiasm. Treat clients as individuals—what works with one may not work with another.

Plan frequent visibility to retie the connection. Attend a client's business and social events when invited. Track your client's work. Attend a trial, even when it's not expected. Send relevant articles and your information newsletter. Remember birthdays and send thank-you notes. Small thoughtful actions will reap huge rewards.

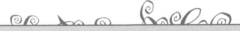

Wizard's Tip: Make your client the hero. Remember Peter Pan and Tinkerbell? When she spread her pixie dust, he got the benefit. When a project goes well, give your clients credit for the success. They'll love you for it.

10 WAYS TO RETIE THE CONNECTION

1. Send follow-up thank-you letters.
2. Send information newsletters.
3. Send articles on latest trends in healthcare.
4. Ask for feedback on reports.
5. Drop by the office.
6. Speak at legal conferences.
7. Write and send out news releases.
8. Inquire about the outcome of cases.
9. Offer to present an in-service.
10. Send gifts or cards for special occasions.

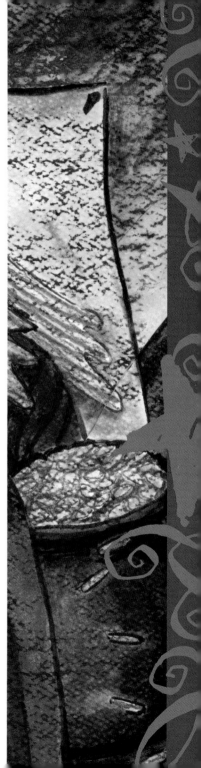

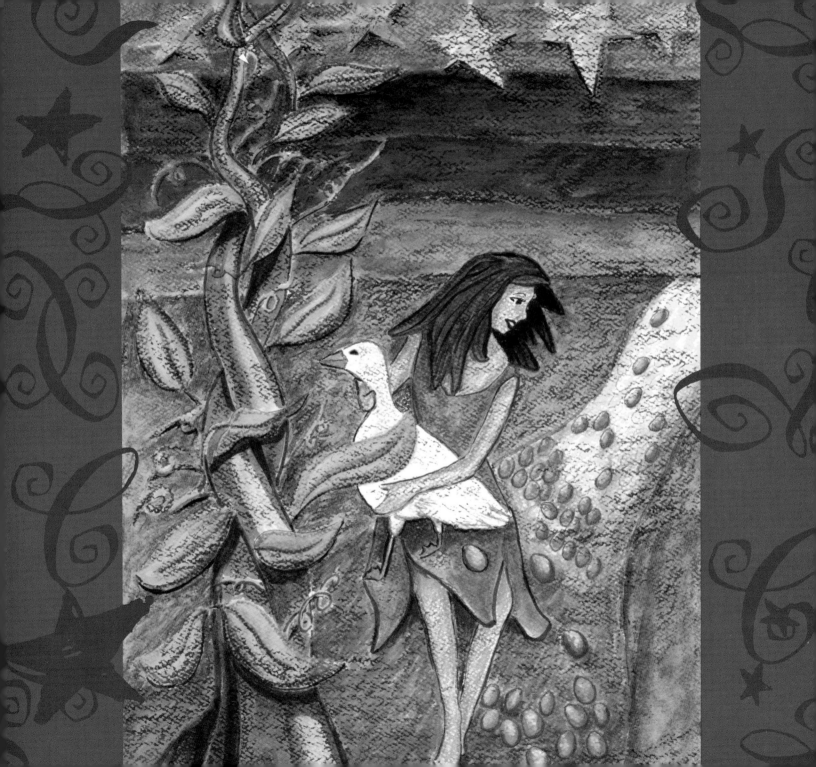

BE A SORCERER OF SALES

When Jack traded his cow for a handful of magic beans, he made a significant sale. The old woman got the cow, which was a valuable commodity, and Jack got the seeds that grew a wondrous beanstalk, where he discovered an enchanted goose that laid fabulous golden eggs. Jack and the old woman both walked away winners. The most successful sales begin with the amazingly simple concept of win-win.

The great sales wizard Zig Ziglar tells us we can get anything we want if we help enough other people get what they want. Put on your sorcerer's hat, your conjurer's cloak, your ruby slippers and charm your attorney-prospects with the spells, potions and elixirs in this powerful section.

You'll discover the magic words to tame the Gatekeeper Dragon and reject the Rejection Ogre.

You will overcome any fears as you sell your magical CLNC® services to attorneys. You'll start your own collection of fabulous golden eggs.

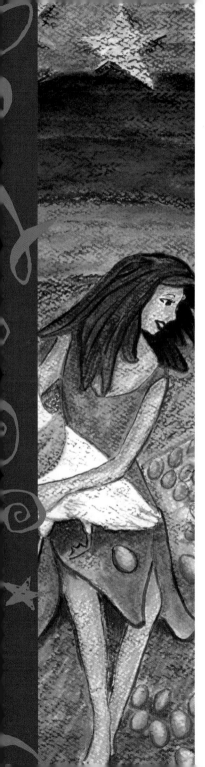

DRESS FOR SUCCESS WITH NOTHING UP YOUR SLEEVES

When casting a spell in the privacy of her office, a proper wizard wouldn't be caught levitating without her purple cloak, pointed hat and those elusive ruby slippers. To cast powerful spells with attorney-prospects and clients, and at networking events, your cloak, hat and slippers will look considerably different, but must be equally effective.

ASSEMBLE YOUR SORCERER'S CHARMS:

* Your power suit—preferably blue, gray, black or camel
* Conservative makeup (women wizards only)
* A flattering hairstyle with a professional cut
* A leather briefcase or portfolio
* A professional-looking pen and presentation folder

OPTIONAL ELIXIRS:

A personal image consultant—many department stores offer the service free

A Montblanc pen

Power up your image using every resource at your disposal to look like you've already made it to the top of your profession. Invest in the best quality suit (you only need one), shoes and briefcase. You'll cast more powerful spells with one proper wizard suit than with a closet full of inferior muggle garb. After all, you can wear only one at a time. Three smart blouses or shirts and ties and you have all the wizard costumes you'll need.

Gold, silver or pearl jewelry in a classic design always looks professional on women wizards. Invest in an expensive-looking watch.

Shoes should be conservative—no sandals or spike heels. Buy good quality. Polish your shoes and check for scuffed toes and worn heels every time you wear them.

Immaculate grooming is imperative—including a manicure. Brush and press your suit between dry cleanings. Women wizards should carry an extra pair of panty hose in the glove compartment and a bottle of clear nail polish for quick repairs.

From head to toe, every detail counts.

Now combine your sorcerer's charms with your mirror of confidence.

MY NEXT POWER-IMAGE INVESTMENT IS

_____

_____

_____

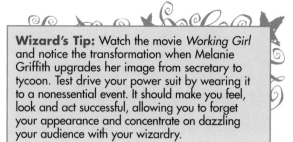

Wizard's Tip: Watch the movie *Working Girl* and notice the transformation when Melanie Griffith upgrades her image from secretary to tycoon. Test drive your power suit by wearing it to a nonessential event. It should make you feel, look and act successful, allowing you to forget your appearance and concentrate on dazzling your audience with your wizardry.

A sample spell that worked magic

A friend shared that when she started her marketing business she wore clothes that looked good but were not traditional business attire. She received compliments but not many sales. When she changed to a conservative power suit, her sales increased 500% immediately, with no other change in her presentation.

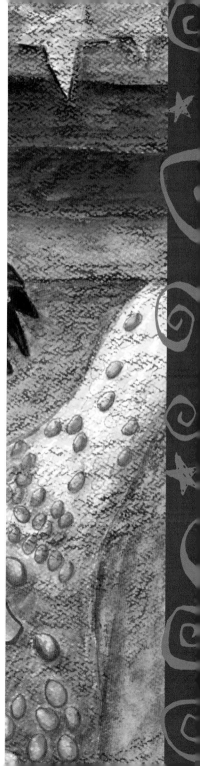

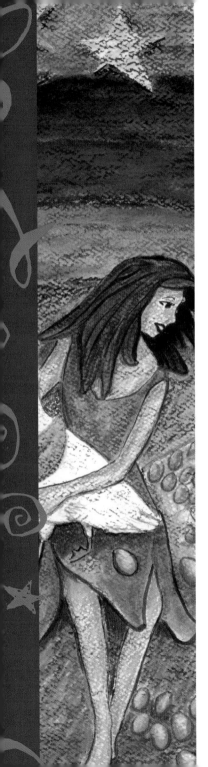

OVERCOME YOUR FEARS OF ENTERING THE ATTORNEY DRAGON'S LAIR

Every wizard harbors anxiety about certain aspects of entrepreneurship. This is the time you long to pull your invisibility cloak over your head and hide. The fact that fear is universal doesn't make it any easier to face, but the following elixir will enable you to vanquish your most dreaded demons and send them to the dungeon where they belong.

PREPARE YOUR ELIXIR WITH:

* Comfortable conjuring clothes
* Encouraging music
* A porcupine quill and dragon's blood for writing

Naming your fear is the first step in conquering it. Are you afraid an attorney will say no, I don't need your services? Pose a question you are not comfortable with or don't know how to answer? Name your three big fears and write them down.

Ask yourself, "What is the worst that could happen?"

Determine your best response to each situation. Evaluate alternatives.

Practice your response until you're comfortable. Create a CLNC® action plan for facing your first dragon.

Wizard's Tip: Summoning the courage to overcome fear in any part of your life will help you conquer your fear in other areas. Refuse to allow anxiety to paralyze your actions. Approach the attorney dragon professionally. Talk about what you do. Bring it up in casual conversation or approach a sensitive topic directly. Ignore any flashing eyes and fiery breath—they're probably just for show—and listen objectively to the dragon's roar. Formulate the appropriate positive response. Deliver it firmly and coolly, in your most wizardly manner.

A SAMPLE SPELL THAT WORKS MAGIC

* Write about accomplishments you've achieved that you were once afraid to tackle.
* Write down one thing in any part of your life that you're afraid to do—skydive, rock climb, exhibit at a legal conference.
* Make your action plan to tackle it now.
* Although I'm afraid, I will _____ on _____ (date).
* Celebrate conquering your fear.

Polish Your Confidence in the Magic Mirror

"Mirror, mirror on the wall, who's the most confident Certified Legal Nurse Consultant℠ of them all?" You are, of course, if you cast this magic spell.

Start your incantation with:

* Preparation—know your material
* Research—know your prospects' background
* Confident posture—chin up, back straight, shoulders and hips parallel
* Confident voice—strong, low and deliberate
* Confident handshake—firm but not crushing
* Your most enchanting smile
* Your interview script
* Your *I Am a Successful CLNC® Success Journal*
* Affirmations

Optional elixir:

Confidence-building CDs by your favorite motivational wizards

Practice your interview script until you can ask and answer questions without looking at notes. Be completely rehearsed when you ask for the sale. Practice in front of your magic mirror and notice your facial expressions. Role-play with a friend, family member, mentor or a CLNC® colleague.

Review pertinent material just before going to a sales, business or networking event including any research you've done on the organization or prospect.

Revisit your skills and talents by browsing through your *CLNC® Success Journal*.

Warm up your voice on the way to the event by reciting out loud, "I am a successful CLNC® consultant," and your other favorite affirmations. Exaggerate your voice, roll it, shout, whisper.

Arrive early and freshen up. Don't let them see you sweat. Project confidence. Think of something positive and humorous. Stand and walk as if a string holds your head, spine, hips and feet in a single, comfortably straight line. Make eye contact and remember to smile.

Finally, make them an offer they can't refuse.

> **Wizard's Tip:** Confidence is a cloak you can wear no matter how many butterflies flutter inside you. Preparation gives you inner confidence. Appearance gives you outer confidence. When you stand, walk, smile and shake hands in a confident manner, your audience assumes you are at ease. And magically, your cloak of confidence, along with your preparation, makes you feel as if you could enchant the world.

A confidence enchantment that doesn't fade in the mirror

* Mirror check—Is your hem or tie straight? No spinach or lipstick on your teeth?
* Materials check—Briefcase orderly? Pertinent files inside? Did you remember your pen and notepad?
* Calendar check—Are you headed for the right place at the right time?

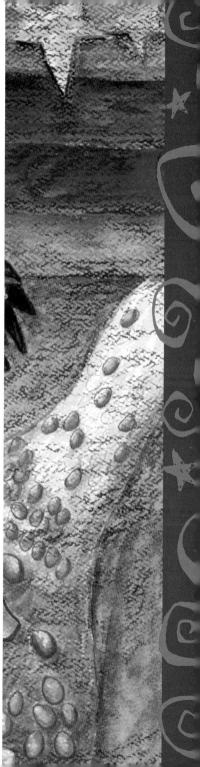

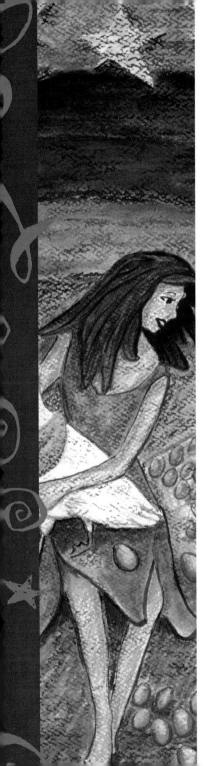

HEAT UP
YOUR COLD CALLS

Dorothy gathered a trio of courageous friends on her way to make the biggest cold call of all—asking the great Wizard of Oz for a favor. In contrast, *you* are the wizard calling on prospects to do *them* a favor—provide excellent advice that will help them win their medical-related cases. Friends like Scarecrow, Lion and Tin Man can magically turn your cold calls warm by making referrals and introductions. Always follow up promptly. Meanwhile, work your own magic—dial, smile and bewitch.

GATHER YOUR MAGICIAN'S TOOLS:

* A long list of prospects—50 to 200 names
* A script customized to the attorney-prospect you plan to call
* A specific name of who to contact within the firm
* A scheduled time to make calls
* A list of frequently asked questions and your answers
* Brochures, business cards and introductory letters ready to mail on request
* A mirror

Warm up your voice before making the first call. Heat up your attitude by first phoning someone who will welcome your call—not a casual friend, but a favorite client, if possible, or a fellow wizard. Warm up your smile in the mirror.

Establish common ground quickly by stating where you met, or mention someone you know in common or an association to which you both belong. If none of that is possible,

give a positive reason why this person's name leapt out at you as an attorney who will benefit from your CLNC® services.

Get to the point in 30 seconds.

Answer questions confidently and succinctly. If the questions keep coming, suggest "getting together" to talk face to face. Avoid using the word "appointment."

> **Sorcerer's Tip:** A wizard of sales hears the word "no" and never takes it personally. The prospect is simply not ready—yet. Maybe later. Cold calling is a numbers game. You'll call seven names on average to get one person to talk to you. Don't let the six who are "not yet ready" keep you from calling the one who wants and needs your special kind of CLNC® magic. The more cold calls you make, the more interviews you'll get and the more chances to transform prospects into clients. Dial, smile, bewitch and ring up sales.

Power words that work magic

According to a Yale University study, the following 12 words are the most powerful in the English language. Build them into your script. Keep this list handy during your cold calls. Use them appropriately and often.

1. You
2. Save
3. Results
4. Health
5. Love
6. Proven
7. Money
8. New
9. Easy
10. Safety
11. Guaranteed
12. Discovery

3 steps to a selling presentation

1. Introduce yourself—your name and your company name.
2. State an opening benefit that gives the prospect a reason to listen. Ask yourself why the prospect should take time out of a busy day to respond to your call. Example: *Attorneys are recognizing that using a Certified Legal Nurse Consultant*^{CM} *to evaluate the medical issues in a case gives the attorney a competitive advantage.*
3. Confirm a "time to sit down together." Ask to schedule a time for you and the attorney to meet regarding the benefits of using a Certified Legal Nurse Consultant^{CM}. Give the prospect specific choices. Example: a) immediately, or b) Thursday afternoon at 2:00pm.

Opening Statements to Avoid

These openers lack confidence.

Sorry to bother you...

I thought I might call to see...

Could I have a few minutes of your time?

An apologetic opening statement does not instill confidence or inspire action. A benefit statement gets the attorney's attention and sparks interest. Always ask yourself, what's in it for them?

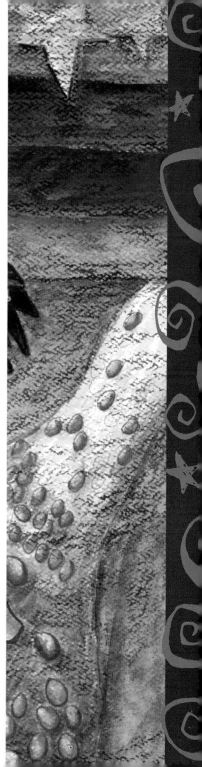

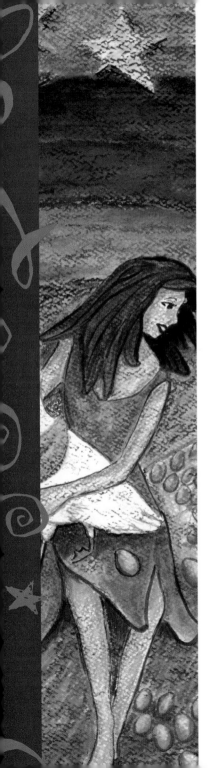

Tame the Gatekeeper Dragon

Fire-breathing and fierce, the secretary dragon guards the prospect's lair. You'll need powerful charms to finesse your way past. Use this potion and the dragon will not only step aside but will swing the door wide for your grand entrance.

Start your magic spell with:

* A cup of courage
* An ounce of cleverness
* Lavish amounts of honey

Optional elixir:

The classic *How to Win Friends and Influence People* by Dale Carnegie

Approach the dragon on a personal level, with respect and interest. Politely introduce yourself. Compliment the dragon, directly or indirectly—"Bill mentioned that John really relies on you," or "I've heard your firm is one of the best."

Drop a referral name, if you have one. "John's colleague Mrs. Miller referred me…"

Build a relationship. Be kind, be thoughtful.

Enlist the dragon's help—"I'm having difficulty with…reaching Mr. Smith…I understand you're the person who can…(e.g., tell me the best time to call back)."

Whether you charm your way past or not, send a thank-you card—"I appreciate your time…" Make notes and call again in two weeks.

If your charm is failing you, draw on your courage and wits. Send a letter to the attorney stating that you will call. When the dragon answers, say, "Mr. Grant is expecting my call…" If asked what the call is about, say, "…regarding a review of medical records."

Continue to build a relationship with the gatekeeper. Pay attention to cues that tell you what the dragon appreciates or enjoys. Give small, appropriate gifts such as chocolates, flowers or a magical object for the desk.

> **Wizard's Tip:** The gatekeeper dragon is doing a job, not attacking you personally. Beneath all the scales and fearsome roar beats a heart. Touch the heart, befriend the dragon, and that breath of fire will burn a path for your success.

A sample spell to reach the unreachable

* Ask the person answering the phone which hours the attorney is usually in the office.
* Call in the early morning, during lunch or after 5:00pm, when the dragon is not there.
* Send an information newsletter.

Never Interview Without Your Ruby Slippers

Dorothy, wearing her best smile and her ruby slippers, finally gets to see the great wizard. He has a big loud voice and looms threateningly. He tells her to go away. Like Dorothy, you are persistent, patient and courageous. You expect rejection, because that's an attorney's nature, and you ignore it. You enchant, you mesmerize, you turn barriers into an opportunity to build value.

Start your magic spell with:

* Your 30-second introduction—including the attorney benefit
* Your interview script—including answers to the common questions and possible objections
* Your most confident smile
* Your qualifications and experience
* Your dazzling enthusiasm
* Your business cards and brochures
* A sample work product
* A letter of recommendation
* An ounce of indifference

Approach the attorney with an attitude of peer-level respect. The attorney is a professional; you are a professional—each in your own discipline.

Keep your objective firmly in mind: introduce the attorney to the benefits of hiring you.

Be succinct and enthusiastic about your abilities. Provide examples of situations in which you have and can help win cases.

Express an interest in the attorney's practice.

Ask for the business—"Which cases on your desk now would benefit from a CLNC® consultant's opinion?"

Mention your risk-free guarantee.

Play your cards one at a time—introduction, qualifications, experience and sample work product—deliberately, with courage, enthusiasm and your most enchanting smile.

Offer to do a first screening at a one-time reduced rate—but only when you feel certain it's the only way you'll leave with a case to review.

My next interview is with

_____

Wizard's Tip: Practice first on an attorney you have no desire to work with and see if you can walk away with a case to review. The first interview is practice. Behind his smoke and mirrors, the great Oz was a kindly, crafty old trickster. So are most attorneys.

An elixir to listen to

Create a recording of yourself enthusiastically overcoming barriers and responding to the most frequent objections. Listen to it frequently and always review it just before each interview.

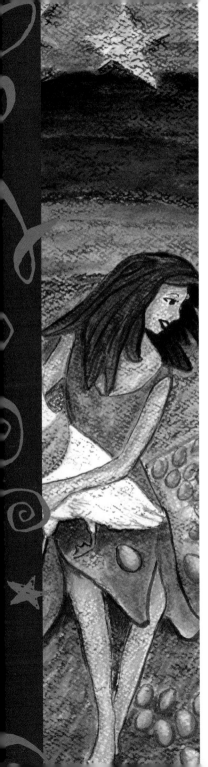

 # Reject the Rejection Ogre

Shrek the ogre would never have found his one true love if he had not finally gotten up the nerve to risk rejection and tell her how he felt. They were made for each other, yet could have gone through life never knowing it. You are the perfect match for a number of attorneys who desperately need a Certified Legal Nurse Consultant^{CM}, but how will you know until you meet? How will you meet unless you're willing to risk rejection? Patience, enthusiasm, courage and persistence—use this potion to boost the power of your magic charms and to reject for yourself the attorneys who are not right for you.

Start your magic rejection potion with:

* A box of tissue
* A shoulder to cry on
* A glass of your favorite soothing beverage
* A box of chocolates or cauldron cakes
* A tantalizing trash novel
* A good night's sleep
* An attitude of gratitude

Optional elixir:

The TNT Network DVD, *Door to Door*, with William H. Macy

When a door is slammed in your face—literally or figuratively—you simply knock on the next door. After a day of slammed doors, however, you might need time out for a pity party. Take five minutes to unload your problems on a fellow CLNC® wizard, who will know how to respond, and another five minutes to cry on a sympathetic shoulder. Then get over it. Get a good night's sleep and wake up ready to knock on the next 20 doors.

Read your affirmations.

Keep in mind that the attorney who said "no" is just one of 1,143,358* prospects. You have 1,143,357 more attorneys who might say "yes." Have ready a long list of prospects—50 to 200—and move on to the next one.

Recognize that it's not about you. The attorney is not rejecting you personally, but simply doesn't yet recognize the need for your CLNC® services.

Review your strategy for turning that "no" into a "yes."

Recognize also that it's just a "no" for now. Eventually, every attorney who needs the magic you can bring to winning a case will seek your assistance.

Invoke your attitude of gratitude for the opportunity to be told "no."

My next prospects are

_____

_____

*Compiled by: American Bar Association, Market Research Department.

The number 30

One study in the psychology of sales tells us that:

- 30% of the people we meet are *immediate* decision makers. If you make a good presentation, and the prospect needs what you're selling, the sale happens.
- 30% are *repetition-based* decision makers. Ask that person, "how many times would I have to show you I'm good at what I do," and he will answer two, three, four, five or maybe 20, and that answer tells you exactly how many times you need to make a professional contact before he is comfortable buying.
- 30% are *time-based* decision makers. If asked the same question, they will not reply with a number at all, but will say, "two weeks," or "six months." That precise amount of time must pass before the person feels comfortable making a decision.

We cannot expect to sell to these time-based and repetition-based buyers on the first contact. No matter how terrific your presentation, they're not comfortable making a decision.

> **Wizard's Tip:** Statistics tell us that sales is a numbers game. You may have to call on 20 attorneys before one finally recognizes your magic as a valuable and much needed service. Invoke the power of your four charms—patience, enthusiasm, courage and persistence. Remember, you only need two or three attorneys to keep you busy full time. Reject rejection. Don your most powerful wizard's hat, make one more phone call, knock on one more door, until you get to "yes."

The number 7

The average number of contacts with one individual before a buying decision is made is seven.

1. Start with an introductory letter, then follow that with a telephone call. That's two contacts.
2. Perhaps the prospect is not ready to commit and says to call again in a couple of weeks. Take the opportunity to send a thank-you note for the time spent on the phone and verify that you will follow up in two weeks. That makes three contacts.
3. When you phone again, that's four contacts.
4. If the prospect agrees to a meeting, that's five contacts—and you might make a sale.

   But what if his magic number is seven? You made a great presentation, but he doesn't have a case right now. You go home feeling defeated.
5. After the five-minute pity party and five-minute cry, send a thank-you letter for the time you spent together. Briefly remind the prospect of a specific CLNC® service, mention again your risk-free guarantee and say you will call again in a few weeks. That's six contacts.
6. Send your information newsletter. That's seven contacts.
7. When you telephone in a few weeks, perhaps you make a sale. If not, simply say you will stay in touch. His magic number might be 14. Or perhaps he needs six months.

In any case, your information newsletter will arrive periodically, and you will follow up with phone calls. Eventually, with your wizardly charm and excellent follow-through, you'll make a sale. It's just a numbers game.

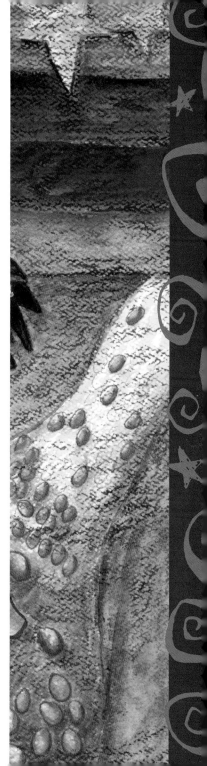

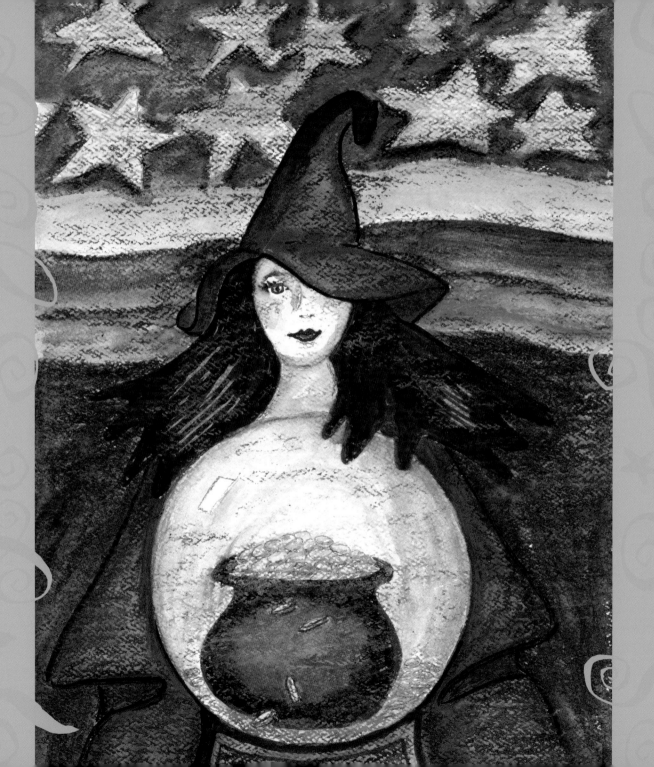

Profit from Your Fortune-Telling Powers

The ultimate reward of being your own boss is financial, physical, mental, spiritual and emotional freedom. However, like King Midas, you might turn everything you touch to gold and still end up bereft of the important aspects of success. Financial wizardry releases the power in you to forecast your own success while enjoying and enriching the relationships that contribute to that success.

Peek into your crystal ball, practice your sleight-of-hand, then use the spells and potions in this insightful section to spin straw into gold. Discover the magic formula for increasing your financial reward and enhancing your lifestyle while ensuring continuous growth of your CLNC® business. Ride your magic carpet over the rainbow and secure your pot of gold—your investment in your future. Then practice the sorcery of brilliant budgeting, clever negotiating and skillful managing to create prosperity for yourself, your CLNC® subcontractors, and every pixie, elf and genie in your circle of influence.

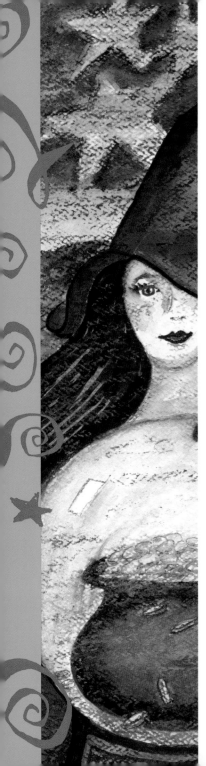

Equip Your Wizard's Workshop with a Brilliant Budget

How does a magician pay for all those birds that materialize only to fly off into the audience? Does a wizard's budget sheet include a column for escaped rabbits? Or top hats soiled by rabbit pellets? Business is often a constantly changing obstacle course, and while some people let the obstacles slow them down, others see the obstacles as stepping stones. When you use the following spell, your budget becomes a stepping stone to bigger and better business adventures.

Start your magic spell with:

★ An office inventory listing equipment, supplies, phones and reference materials
★ A list of routine business expenses—marketing, office expenses, CLNC® subs
★ Your salary based on personal expenses
★ Your hourly rate for CLNC® wizard's services
★ A list of "needs"
★ A list of "really wants"

Optional elixir:

Software for business finance, such as QuickBooks®

Determine the magic number. This is what you must earn each month to meet your total expenses. Don't forget to include income and sales taxes, health and disability insurance and an investment in your future—an IRA or SEP account. A rule of thumb is that you will need to earn at least one-third more as an independent business owner than you did as an employee to realize the same salary.

Identify any purchases you will make in the next year, including marketing materials, office equipment and special elixirs.

Based on your hourly rate, determine how many hours you will need to invoice each week to meet expenses, including paying yourself a salary.

My brilliant monthly budget is

$ _____

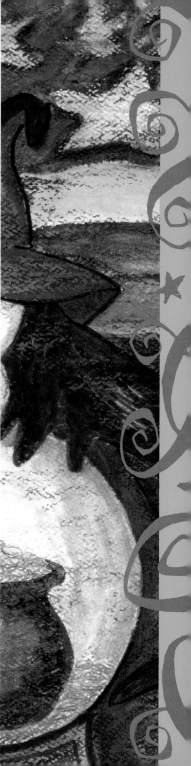

SAMPLE EXPENSES FOR A CLNC® WIZARD

- Marketing—10% of Gross

  During the start-up phase you can expect marketing costs to draw against a higher percentage of your gross earnings. Project the total over the year to find the exact percentage.

- Payroll—70% of Gross

  Entrepreneurs often discover that they cannot draw a personal salary during the first three to six months of doing business.

In this start-up phase, you may need to rely on savings or a second income. Payroll, including your own salary, should not exceed 70% of gross earnings.

- Overhead—20% of Gross

  Include in overhead expense: your phone line, Internet service, accounting services, legal services, subcontractors, insurance, licenses and permits, consumable supplies, taxes, repairs, maintenance, dues, subscriptions and fees.

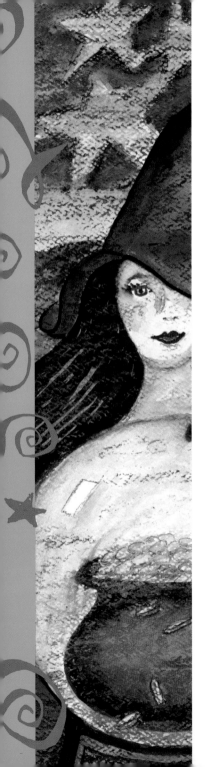

Negotiate a Wizard's Fee

Your time is valuable, and even the strongest magic cannot replace it. Determining a fair price that rewards you generously for your knowledge, wizardry and experience will prepare you to approach the topic of fees successfully and with confidence.

Assemble the alchemy:

* A cup of self-worth
* A pixie-dust list of your accomplishments
* A dash of win-win attitude
* A seductive goal such as a car, house or vacation with pictures to inspire you
* Your fee mantra, "My fee is $____"
* A sample script for stating your fee
* A sample contract or letter agreement
* A book on the sorcery of negotiation
* A magic mirror

Prepare your mind-set by reading wonder-working passages from a book on negotiation. Scan the sample contract or letter agreement. Set these items aside.

Stir your cauldron of confidence by reviewing your abilities, accomplishments and inspirational pictures.

Jot down your bottom-line professional fee (no less than $125.00 an hour). This is your walk-away. No matter how enchanting the job, if it doesn't pay at least this amount it's not the job for you.

Jot down your preferred fee—a devilish amount that rewards you fairly and generously.

Once you have these two figures, practice by saying, "My fee is $___" in your magic mirror.

Rehearse with a CLNC® colleague, friend or your magic mirror, so that when you meet with attorney-prospects you can smile, wave a mental wand and present your fee incantation with mesmerizing confidence.

Alchemist's Secret: A reporter once asked J. Paul Getty if the value of his holdings was indeed a billion dollars. Getty responded, "I suppose so. But remember, a billion dollars doesn't go as far as it used to." A big step in levitating from employee to entrepreneur is to learn to think like an entrepreneur. Compared to your hourly rate in the nursing profession, your consulting fee might sound high to you. Instead, consider your fee in comparison to other professionals. What do psychologists make per hour? Dermatologists? Your CPA? Your attorney-prospects? Meditating briefly on these amounts should put your own fee in perspective.

My CLNC® fee is $_____

"Mirror, mirror on the wall, I am worth this fee after all."

Negotiate Your Contracts to Spin Straw into Gold

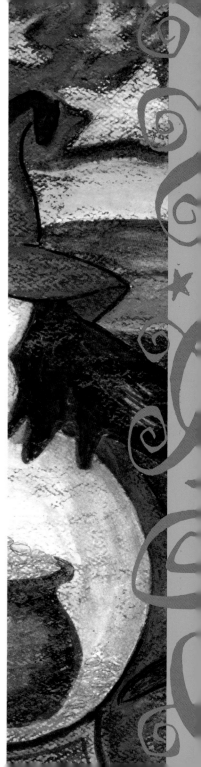

When the king instructed the miller's daughter to spin straw into gold, Rumplestiltskin instantly got the upper hand. The wicked little gnome had the skill and knowledge the girl lacked. To gain his magical services, she had to give up her ring, her necklace and her first-born child. As a Certified Legal Nurse Consultant[CM] you, however, already know how to spin straw into gold. Use your skills and this potion to negotiate your contracts, and you'll never have to give up a single cherished possession.

Start your contracts potion with:

* A sample contract from *e-Contracts! Contracts! Contracts!*
* Your power suit
* A win-win attitude
* Your four charms—courage, enthusiasm, patience and persistence

Assess your bargaining position on a point *before* you address that point with the other side. Set the pace of negotiations by getting your ideas on paper and writing a rough draft of the contract. Make a list of what you want from the relationship. Check your draft against the list. Think like a clever, realistic gnome: try to imagine what could go wrong, and then address that possibility.

After your own attorney has looked at the contract, send a copy to your attorney-client.

Write in plain English. Keep it simple. Many contracts are one to two pages. Put everything in writing.

Always negotiate from a position of comfort—your power suit, your wizard's robe, whatever makes you feel magical.

Listen carefully. Sometimes we miss what people are telling us. Let them explain. If you don't understand a term, don't agree to it. Get the other side to put what it means in writing.

Always ask for more than you want or expect—you might be surprised to get it!

Speak and act with confidence. Look your attorney-client in the eye and think everything through. Don't be in a hurry to agree, but don't say "no" right away. Be magically, confidently flexible. You don't have to win every point.

> **Sorcerer's Secret:** Remember, if you don't ask, the answer is always no. Summon your magic charm of courage. Refuse to be afraid to ask for what you want, and don't give away your first-born child.

A sample spell that works magic

Commit to become a contract wizard with e-Contracts! Contracts! Contracts!

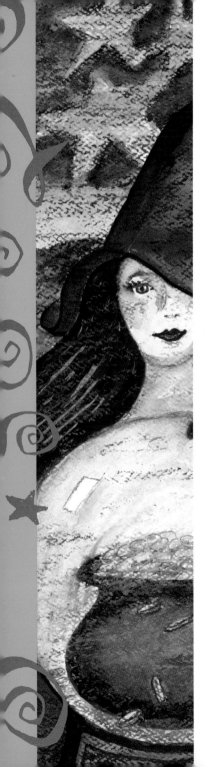

Make Money Appear with Sleight-of-Hand

Magic is an illusion. While one hand sprinkles the pixie dust and waves the wand, the other hand finesses the trick. To pull a rabbit out of the hat, the magician must execute the sleight-of-hand one, two, three—all in good order. Likewise, while one side of your business handles sales and delivery, the other side takes care of collections. The art of getting paid in a timely manner lies in performing your billing finesse like any good magician—one, two, three, all in good order.

Start your legerdemain with:

* A proper fee negotiation
* An agreed-on budget for the case
* A retainer of 50% to 100%
* An invoice template that includes case name, CLNC® services rendered, rate, itemized expenses, balance due and payment terms
* Expense receipts
* Envelopes and postage

Optional elixir:

Software for tracking time and generating invoices

Prime your billing finesse by building winning relationships. Include open communication regarding fees with your client and your client's office staff. An attorney who pays on time is as good as King Midas.

> **Wizard's Wisdom:** Develop a monthly billing system and practice it faithfully. Never wait until the end of a big project to send your bill. You can bill in regular increments as the case work proceeds. Schedule a specific day to practice making money appear: itemize your expenses, compute your time and post the invoice—one, two, three, like any good magician, all in good order.

The tools of alchemy

Software, such as TimeSlips® *and* QuickBooks.®

Grow Your Hourly Fee Faster than Jack's Beanstalk

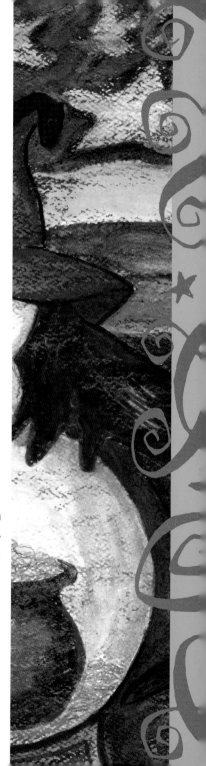

You've invested your magic beans to grow a wondrous beanstalk, and you've captured a few enchanted geese. Yet, the golden eggs fail to cover that exotic vacation and new house you want to build. How do you increase the number of eggs the geese lay? The simple answer is to increase your fees fairly and regularly. When it's time for your fee increase, the following potion works magic.

Begin your incantation with:

* The right fee to start with
* A calendar and the annual date you will increase your fee (5% minimum)

Increase your hourly rate again when you have more business than you and your CLNC® subcontractors can handle. A higher rate might reduce the number of attorneys who use your services, but don't count on it. Higher fees magically tend to indicate that your value has also increased.

Implement smaller incremental adjustments instead of large, infrequent or sporadic increases.

Charge new attorney-clients the higher rate while allowing current clients a grace period before the new rate takes effect. Send advance notice of the impending rate change to your clients, and let them know they're getting the current, lower fee for a specific time period.

Create a script for disclosing the new rate to current attorney-clients, and post the new fee schedule by the phone for your reference when talking to prospects.

Offer a discount to attorney-clients who guarantee a certain number of hours each month. Make sure you communicate to the attorney that they're getting a special deal.

My new fee of $_____ takes effect _____ (date)

> **Shaman's Secret:** Honor and value yourself and your time, and your clients will respect you. When the golden eggs cease to add up to the magic number and a fee increase becomes necessary, don't agonize over it or apologize for it. Just do it.

A magically written incantation

Dear (Client):

I consider you a most valued client and appreciate the business we've conducted together over the past months. Finding it necessary to increase my hourly rate, I offer you a special consideration. Although new clients will pay a rate of $_____ , your firm will see no fee increase for the next three months. Any work contracted after that period will be invoiced at the new rate. I value your business and look forward to working with you in the future.

P.S. If you would like to lock in the current fee for an extended time period, perhaps we can negotiate a guaranteed number of hours per month that will benefit both of us.

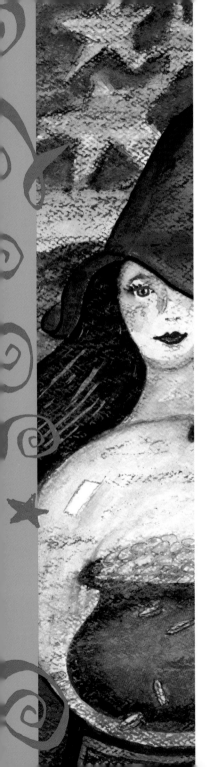

Harness Your Midas Touch to Fill Your Pot with Gold

Like a leprechaun's lucky charm, your money, placed in a magic pocket, attracts more money. Your magic pockets reside in banks, in savings organizations and in the stock market. Recite the incantation of prosperity—I earn, I attract, I invest, I save—and your pot at the rainbow's end will overflow with gold.

Begin your alchemy with:

* A business checking account
* A business savings account
* An IRA or SEP account
* A business budget
* An emergency stash of three to six months of expenses
* A savings goal
* A CPA

Optional elixirs:

A financial planner or software program to help manage investments

The Courage to Be Rich by Suze Orman

Prepare for wealth by acknowledging that you are motivated to prosper. Envision the dollar amount that excites you. Read one financial magazine or electronic newsletter each month.

Add life insurance to your financial plan.

Pave your yellow brick road with a clear understanding of your present financial picture, and make sure your will is up to date.

Pay yourself first. Place the first 10% of every check into a designated savings account, CD or an IRA or SEP account.

I save $_____ every month

Alchemist's Secret: Keep the money flowing. You'll enrich your life in proportion to the amount you give to others. Never give in order to receive, but know that any contributions will be rewarded. Money that flows freely from the heart enriches the giver and provides the leprechaun's lucky charm for attracting more money.

The 80-10-10 Formula for Prosperity

Divide your pot of gold—80% of your earnings, after business expenses, for living, 10% for savings and 10% for tithing.

Enjoy a Lifetime of Golden Eggs

When Jack climbed his magic beanstalk and found the goose who laid golden eggs, he thought his future was mint perfect. He might have been right if only he'd treasured that goose as much as the eggs. Prosperity begins with valuing yourself and others and using sound financial practices. Use this spell to leverage today's beans into a lifetime of golden eggs.

Start your magic spell with:

* Checking and savings accounts
* A retirement plan
* A growth plan for your CLNC® practice
* Patience, persistence, courage, enthusiasm and confidence

Recognize the value of your CLNC® services and charge appropriately. Don't be lured into low fees thinking they will lead to higher fees later. It's harder to raise the bar after it is set.

Leverage your income by using CLNC® wizards as subcontractors. With two subs and a 50% payout on each, you'll double your income.

Stay abreast of what's happening in the legal nurse consulting profession. Always keep learning, improving your magic and striving for excellence.

Work with quality attorneys who recognize quality in others.

Treat every case as if it's the only one you'll be remembered by, and give as much attention as you did on the first case you ever worked. Focus on the attorney-client from your heart and give your all.

Stay fully engaged in the magical process of doing business. Keep up your billing and marketing. Be persistent. Never impeach your credibility and integrity. Notice the impact you make on the industry, and don't kill the golden goose.

Grant yourself permission to dream your own incredible dreams—not someone else's.

Share the wealth. Give back to your community, your faith, family, friends, fellow CLNC® wizards, pixies, elves and your profession.

Prosperity for me is _____

Fortune-Teller's Tip: Prosperity cannot happen on all levels unless you're willing to grow. Look beyond today's problems. Expect great challenges and great accomplishments, and make love deposits daily in your personal relationships. Work as a CLNC® consultant because you love it. Learn to enjoy all the things you do to grow your practice. Use your four charms—courage, enthusiasm, patience and persistence—to nurture the golden goose.

"Prosperity is experiencing balance in life. It is attaining what we want on a mental, physical, emotional, spiritual and financial level. Prosperity is the natural result of opening our minds to our creative imaginations and being willing to act on our ideas."

—*Ruth Ross*

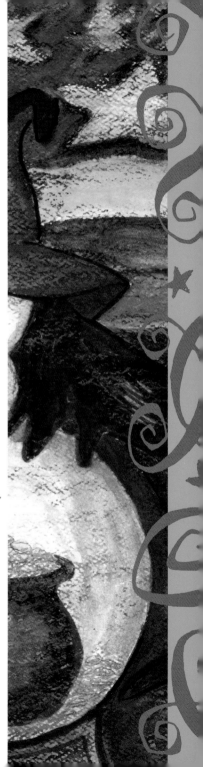

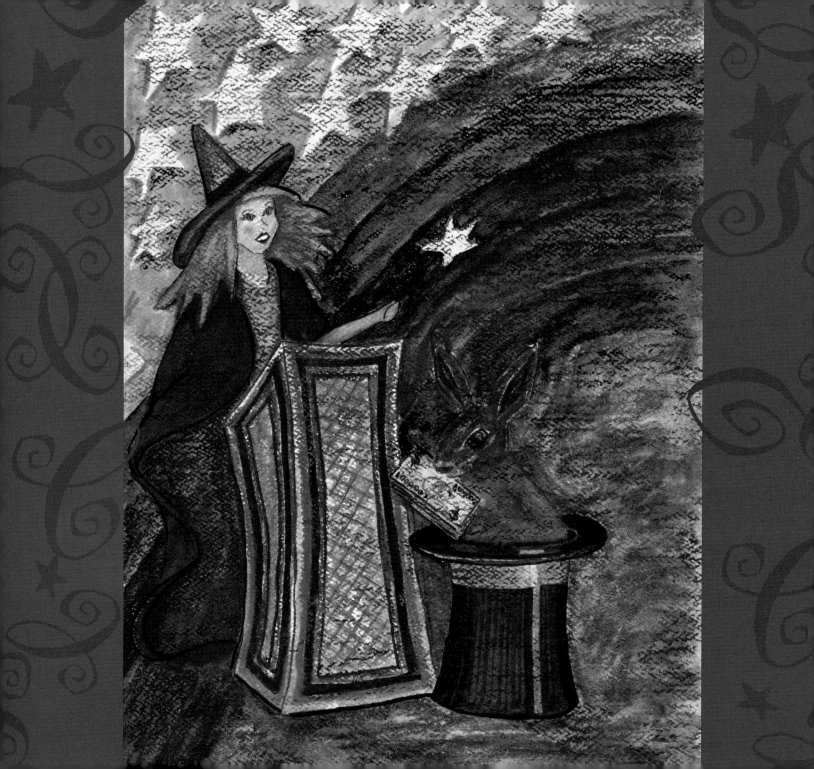

SAY THE MAGIC WORDS

"Rumplestiltskin," murmured the miller's daughter, and at once her misery vanished into the dream life she imagined. Perhaps no one word will be the *open sesame* to your CLNC® dreams, but knowing what to say and when to say it is a talisman to success in any CLNC® venture.

From writing your introductory letter to giving an enchanting talk, you must employ the sorcery of words and let them weave their spell in your CLNC® business.

Use the following potions and elixirs to craft spellbinding communications and to charm your clients with supernatural persuasion. Discover the mesmerizing power of visual, auditory and kinesthetic words. Employ your witching tools—pen and paper, voice mail and email, telephone and lectern—to enchant an audience of one or one thousand. Invoke the elegance of proper etiquette and the meaningful magic of thank you to dot your professional "Is" and cross your wizardly "Ts." *Abracadabra, alakazam*—with intuition, experience and powerful words you bewitch your audience and command your CLNC® future.

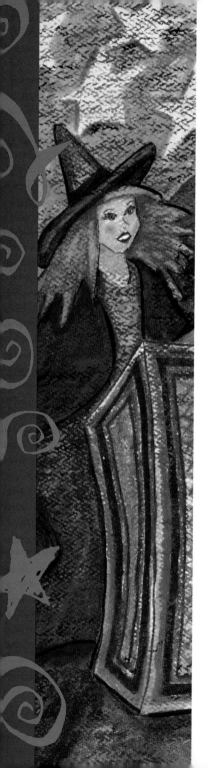

Write with Supernatural Persuasion

"The difference between the right word and the almost right word is the difference between lightning and a lightning bug." —Mark Twain

To cross the bridge and pass the terrible one-eyed troll, the Three Billy Goats Gruff had to be supernaturally persuasive. Persuasive communications are essential in any business, and to write effective communications, you must have a sorcerer's command of grammar and word usage, as well as a lexicon of bewitchingly appropriate phrases. Use this spell to enhance your letters, notes, emails and reports.

Start your communication spell with:

* A word processing program, such as Microsoft Word® or Mac Pages
* A good dictionary
* A thesaurus
* A grammar book
* A style manual or templates for letters and reports

Optional elixir:

***A Grammar Book for You and I...Oops, Me!* by C. Edward Good**

Organize your thoughts before composing your draft. Consider the message you want to deliver and design the communication for your specific audience. If your communication skills, especially grammar and usage, need sharpening, consider taking a business writing course.

Keep it simple; use words everyone will know. Make sure you understand the definition of the words you use, and put them in the right context.

Avoid slang, abbreviations and secret wizard's words. Define medical jargon simply, the way you would before a jury.

Use active voice, not passive.

Active:
* The medical records contained errors.
* A miscommunication caused the wrong dosage administration.

Passive:
* There were errors noted in the medical records.
* The reason he gave the wrong dosage was because of a miscommunication.

Proofread, proofread, proofread. Use automatic spell check on all written communications, and proofread important correspondence and reports at least three times. If you are uncertain, hire a writer or editor to become your second pair of eyes, or buddy up with another wizard whose wisdom you trust.

Sorcerer's Tip: Omit needless words. Avoid a succession of loose sentences. Be clear, be specific and always let the material rest for a while before revising. Fresh eyes catch the wickedest mistakes.

CRAFT CAPTIVATING COMMUNICATION

  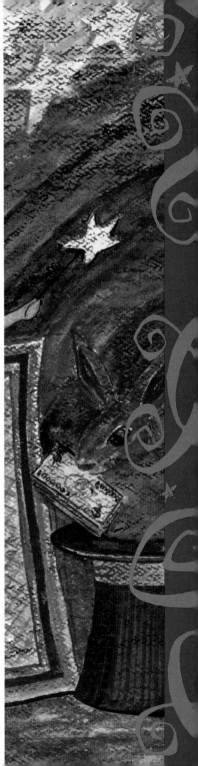

Bubble, bubble, toil and trouble—once said, words cannot be unsaid, and they create their own wizardry as soon as they're spoken. How many times have you said something you wish you hadn't? Certain words can bewitch the mind and ensnare the senses. Use words wisely to charm and enchant as you communicate.

Start your communication charm with:

- ✶ A win-win attitude
- ✶ Positive body language and good posture
- ✶ Direct eye contact—no head tilt
- ✶ Pen or pencil and legal pad for taking notes

Optional elixirs:

Getting to Yes: Negotiating Agreement Without Giving In **by Roger Fisher, Bruce M. Patton and William L. Ury**

Mars and Venus in the Workplace **by John Gray**

Prepare your mind to communicate. Set aside other thoughts and concentrate on the person to whom you are speaking.

If the meeting is at your office, avoid distractions such as pets, kids, phones, magic flutes or braying centaurs.

Listen. Shed your invisibility cloak and show that you are listening by maintaining eye contact, smiling or nodding at appropriate moments. Avoid the constantly bobbing head syndrome.

Acknowledge what you heard, even if you don't agree or can't do it. Restate to clarify.

Think about what you want to say before you say it. Focus on the issue. Be succinct.

Use examples, analogies and brief anecdotes to illustrate complex ideas.

> **Soothsayer's Advice:** Lawyers are bottom line, so don't dawdle. Show that you are alert and interested by your body language and an upbeat tone and pace. Avoid long, run-on sentences. Avoid lengthy diversions. Don't be afraid to consult your prepared notes for the precise words and phrases that will make your point in the most bewitching manner.

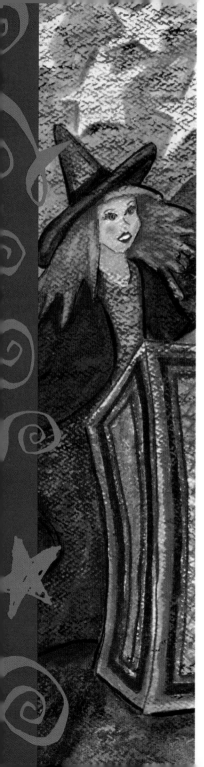

Work Your Spell with the Right Words

Certain words create their own spell. Such words should be collected in jars, stored on a shelf in your wizard's workshop and used selectively. Sorcerers who study communication styles reveal that everyone has three modes: visual, auditory and kinesthetic (feeling). Generally, we favor one communication mode over the others, just as we are predominantly either right- or left-handed.

Let's suppose you are predominantly visual, with kinesthetic as your secondary mode, followed by auditory as the one you use least. If an attorney-prospect is predominantly auditory, you may feel as if you've jumped through the looking glass to have a conversation with the Jabberwock. You and your prospect are speaking two different languages. You can banish this little known but very real problem through the simple magic of awareness and using the right words with the right attorneys.

Start your magic spell with:

* Two open ears
* Two open eyes
* A cup of caring
* A dash of patience
* A heaping dollop of persistence
* Paper and pen
* A phone conversation

Tune in to your prospect, your wizard's ears and eyes alert, and listen for words that reflect the other person's communication mode. Jot down as many words as possible while the attorney is talking. You can then analyze them later.

Visual words include: see, clearly, bright, dull, scenario, reflect, show me, vision, sight, perception, perceive, look at, observe, regard, cast an eye on, get an eyeful, stare, gaze, peek, spy, watch, visualize, inspect, examine, scrutinize, spark and reveal.

Auditory words include: hear, speak, loud, shrill, murmur, call, talk, resounding, tell, inform, overhear, listen, lend an ear to, tell me, bend an ear, eavesdrop, interview, discuss, vouch, converse, chat, say, utter, express, whisper, speak out and clanging.

Kinesthetic words include: walk, move, touch, do, hard, soft, rough, smooth, grab, take, carry, build, fold, get a handle on, give it to me, walk me through it, shoot the breeze, hold, bring out, lay open, point to, press upon, step, lead, go, shatter and earthshaking.

Practice with family and friends. Careful listening will enable you to discover the predominant communication mode of others, which in turn will enable you to communicate more effectively.

Adjust your language to match your attorney-prospect or client. Keep handy a short, secret list of these appropriate words and use them in any conversation. Eventually, you'll become so adept that you won't need your sorcerer's cheat sheet.

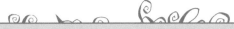

Shaman's Tip: Wizards who rely only on their own predominant communication mode may instantly exempt one-third of all potential prospects. To the attorney, your conversation might seem as strange as Jabberwocky: "'Twas brillig, and the slithy toves did gyre and gimble in the wabe..." Use your word lists—add to them continually—and stretch your style to include all three modes. Place a copy beside the phone; keep one in your portfolio. With practice, you'll magically become more aware and able to charm, bewitch and enchant universally.

DISCOVER YOUR PREDOMINANT COMMUNICATION MODE

Speak into a recorder, describing a vacation experience in detail.

Then replay the recording and list all the visual, auditory and kinesthetic words you hear.

Whichever you use most is your predominant mode.

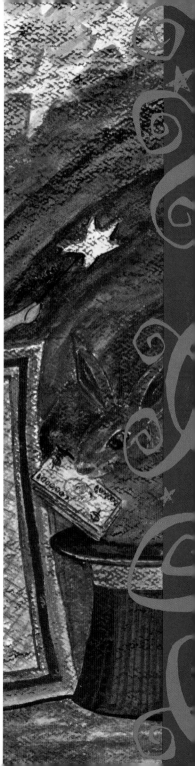

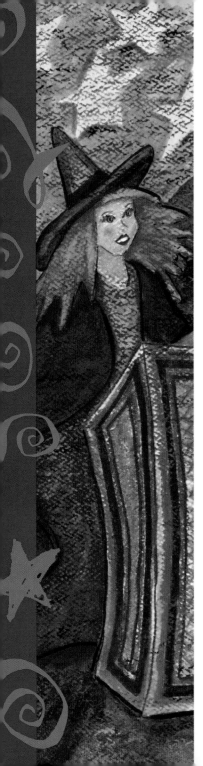

Open Sesame with Your Introductory Letter

When Aladdin approached the cave leading to a wondrous treasure, and found a heavy stone blocking his path, he said the magic words that made the stone slide away. Your *open sesame* to prospective clients begins with your captivating, icebreaking introductory letter. Use this spell and your wizardly charm to write an entrancing letter, then mail it to your list of prospects.

Start your enchantment with:

★ Professional 8½″ x 11″ letterhead with matching #10 envelopes

★ Postage

★ Your prospect list

★ Your most dependable wand

Focus on your prospect—what benefit will she receive from using your magic? Customize the letter to the type of attorney to whom you are writing, and use key words in the first sentence such as, "medical resource," "injury-related lawsuits," "interpret medical records," "health insurance claims" or "dragon's breath burns."

Keep it short—attorneys don't have time to read long-winded letters.

• Introduce yourself and only briefly mention your experience, since your resume will be attached. Focus on your USP and how you will provide benefits no other legal nurse consultant can match.
• Use positive words, such as "advantage" and "benefit."
• Bullet-point your services.

• Suggest you "get together" or "meet in person" for about 15 or 20 minutes. Promise to bring samples of your work.
• State that you will follow up by phone "in a few days," and then do it.
• Include a risk-free guarantee: "If you are not completely satisfied with my work product, notify me in writing within two weeks. I will rework it to your satisfaction or refund your money."

Proofread, proofread, proofread. Set your word processor to automatically spell check, butt dew knot re-lie on spell Czech a loan.

> **Sorcerer's Tip:** Attorneys like doing business with other professionals. Until you meet face to face, your letter represents you. Make sure it looks as professional as you do. Use a conservative business letterhead—save the lavender stationery for personal correspondence. Address the attorney by name. Write in a crisp, upbeat, efficient style and sign your letter in blue ink. This adds a conservative spot of color that gets attention. For an additional bit of bewitchment, put your risk-free guarantee in a P.S. Studies show the P.S. is the part of a letter prospects read first.

Used appropriately, the following words can work magic

Benefit	Opportunity	Certification	Medical terminology
Advantage	CLNC® consultant	Medical-related issues	Healthcare expert

Transform the Phone into a Powerful Bewitching Tool

Like the wand, cauldron, broomstick and computer, the telephone is a powerful witching tool. Used effectively, it collapses space, reduces travel and brings prospects and clients instantly into your office. Use this spell to enhance your telephone magic and enchant callers.

Start your magic spell with:

* A telephone and voice mail
* Your sales script
* A notepad and pen

Optional elixirs:

A headset for keeping your hands free

Maintain a working atmosphere near your phone. Include your sales script, paper and pen and a mirror to reflect your expression. Remember to smile. Put the dog or bird out of earshot before dialing, and let the kids know not to interrupt. Don't eat, chew gum, type or conduct other business—people sense when they don't have your full attention.

Practice your script so that you don't sound as if you're reading it. Keep a list of positive, useful words on hand for responding to questions.

Answer callers with a warm professional voice. State your name or state your company name followed by your name. Listen patiently to the caller's request, without interrupting. Don't let children answer the business line.

> **Wizard's Tip:** Cell phones provide the incredible hocus pocus of allowing you take a broomstick ride to anywhere and still be available as if you're at the office. Set up the voice mail on your cell phone as professionally as on your business line. Turn it off when you're with clients. If it rings while you're talking on your regular office phone, don't answer it. Voice mail will magically take the call.

The sorcery of voice mail

One of the wonder-working devices of your business world is so ordinary that an unsuspecting wizard could easily take it for granted. Set up your voice mail as a marketing tool. First, state your name and company name. Record your greeting along with a brief marketing message that emphasizes your USP. Ask callers to leave a message and a number at which they can be reached. Speak as naturally and warmly as you would answer the phone in person. Give a time frame when you will call back. Keep the message short, simple and free of background noise or static. This is not a time to be cute or to let the elves, pixies or kids chime in. Review your message and update it periodically.

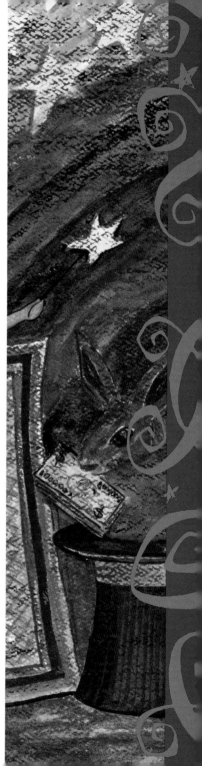

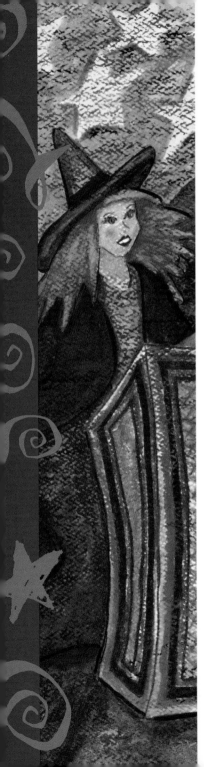

EXPAND YOUR MAGIC POWERS WITH THANK-YOU NOTES

*A**bracadabra! Open sesame! Alakazam!* If asked to name the most powerful phrase, which would you choose? If you said none of the above, you'd get a star on your pointed hat. The most perceptive wizards learn the power of "thank you" before ever stirring a cauldron. Use the following spell to show appreciation and enchant all your prospects and clients.

Start your magic spell with:

★ Professional-looking note cards
★ Your CLNC® Marketing LaunchBox stationery with matching envelopes
★ Postage
★ A wizard's incantation of appreciation

Optional elixir:

The Thank-You Book: Hundreds of Clever, Meaningful and Purposeful Ways to Say Thank You by Robyn Freedman Spizman

Approach the thank-you-note spell as you would any marketing project—with sincerity, purpose and determination. The magic lies in creating a "living" charm that you renew daily.

Consider all the reasons you might want to thank someone in your business:

• Follow up to a phone call—*thank you for the opportunity to visit with you by phone and discuss the advantages of using a Certified Legal Nurse Consultant***CM*...

• Follow up to an interview—*thank you for taking the time to meet with me on (date) so that I could further explain how my legal nurse consulting services will benefit your legal practice*...

• For encouragement—*thank you for those encouraging words last night at the networking meeting*...

• For buying—*I appreciate the opportunity to work with you on (case name).*

• For not buying—*thank you for giving me the opportunity to propose my legal nurse consulting services. While my CLNC® services don't fit your needs at this time, perhaps you'll come upon a case in the future that requires the nursing and healthcare knowledge that I can provide. In any case, I sincerely appreciate being considered.*

Use handwritten notes when possible. Use formal thank-you letters on business letterhead when they need to be longer, or if your handwriting is truly illegible.

Proofread, proofread, proofread.

My next five thank-you notes will go to

1. _____
2. _____
3. _____
4. _____
5. _____

Merlin's Tip: The cleverest wizard will mail out three to five thank-you notes every day, in addition to expressing appreciation verbally and by email. Handwritten notes will help grow your business faster than Jack's magic beans and will help you retain clients like a pair of enchanted golden handcuffs.

Reasons to say thank you

✓ For such a good idea
✓ For retaining my CLNC® services
✓ For referring me
✓ For words of wisdom
✓ For being thoughtful
✓ For help

✓ For the opportunity to consult on such an interesting case
✓ For remembering me
✓ For considering my CLNC® services
✓ For encouragement
✓ For returning my call

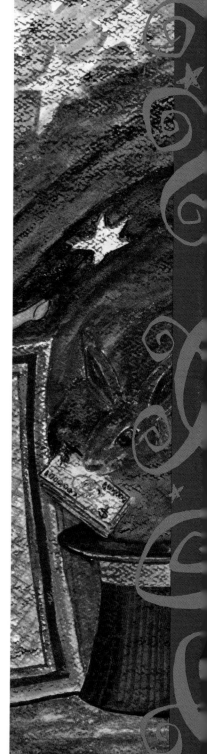

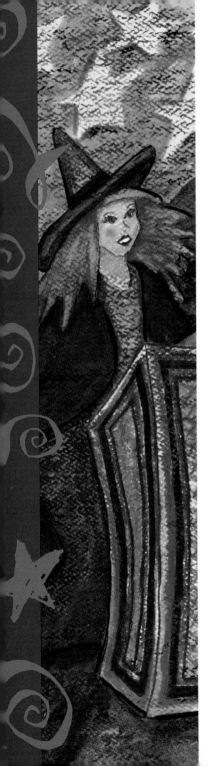

Invoke the Easiest Magic of All— Laughter and Humor

Occasionally a magician has a terrific sense of humor that warms up the audience and makes them want to believe in magic. Humor also keeps the audience misdirected while the magician works his sleight-of-hand. If you have a natural ability to make people laugh, perhaps you can use its spell to break the ice with attorney-prospects, and with clients when all is not well.

Start your magic spell with:

* A sense of humor
* Appropriate jokes
* Quips
* Funny quotations

Optional elixir:

A joke-of-the-day calendar or website

Know your audience. Let the attorney take the lead. If she cracks jokes, then you can feel comfortable following suit. However, keep the humor tasteful. Leave the lawyer jokes at home, and recognize that attorneys might not find dark hospital humor funny.

Be willing to laugh at yourself. The most endearing comedians are the butt of their own jokes. Never make a wisecrack at the expense of your client, prospect, anyone on their staff or a competitor.

Sharpen your sense of humor by reading something funny daily. Post humorous signs near your computer and read them when a project is going poorly or you're feeling cranky.

Collect humorous quotations. Memorize those that might be funny in specific business situations and use them with care.

Humor in your own workplace is a blessing. Laugh every hour, especially when marketing.

> **Sorcerer's Advice:** If you're comfortable with humor, use it. If not, be cautious. When in doubt about a joke or a remark, don't say it. Merlin, Morgana and Dumbledor dropped the occasional quip but were otherwise reserved when speaking.

Weave Spells with Enchantingly Persuasive Talks

Imagine the persuasion techniques the wily tailors used to convince a king he needed a suit of clothes made from magical, invisible cloth. Words weave spells, and weaving a talk that beguiles and persuades your audience takes a special potion like this one.

Start your magic speech potion with:

- ★ A topic of spellbinding interest to attorneys
- ★ A splash of amusing anecdotes
- ★ A sprinkle of intriguing examples
- ★ A dash of startling statistics
  Enthusiasm and courage

Optional elixir:

Secrets of Successful Speakers by Lilly Walters, Lillet Walters and Norman Vincent Peale

Assess your audience. What do they already know? What are their burning questions?

Keep it simple. Your topic should be a small piece of a big idea. You can't teach everything you know in 30 minutes.

Keep it entertaining. We all learn better when the information given is interesting and exciting.

Follow the magic formula: 15% of your time should be devoted to an opening hook, 5% to the closing pitch and 80% to engaging information.

Hook your audience. A captivating, persuasive opening has five parts:

1. The attention getter—a brief anecdote, intriguing example or startling statistic.
2. The link—a one-sentence elaboration linking the hook to the speech.
3. Your credentials—a smooth statement of why you're qualified to give this talk.
4. The preview—the three points you plan to make, quickly stated.
5. The sales trigger lead-in—"If you use the suggestions I give you, I guarantee..." This statement can make the difference between walking away after your talk with business in your pocket—or not.

Deliver three points in the informative body of your talk. Illustrate each point with anecdotes, examples and statistics. Make each memorable with alliteration, acronyms or humor.

Close by looping back to the opening: refer to the attention getter, then restate the link, the three points and the guarantee. "If you use these suggestions, I guarantee you'll..."

My next persuasive talk is to

Wizard's Tip: The best talks are 20% information and 80% delivery. Your reason for speaking is to inform, educate, persuade and sell. If you use the suggestions above, every talk will be informative and effective, and like the wily tailors' magic cloth, your persuasive sales pitch will be invisible.

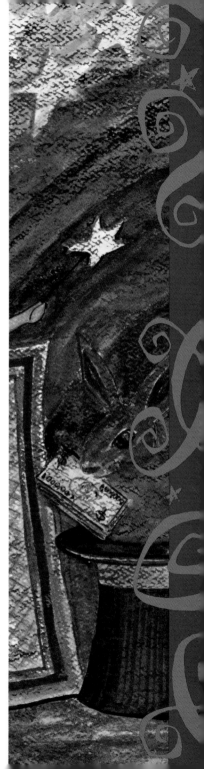

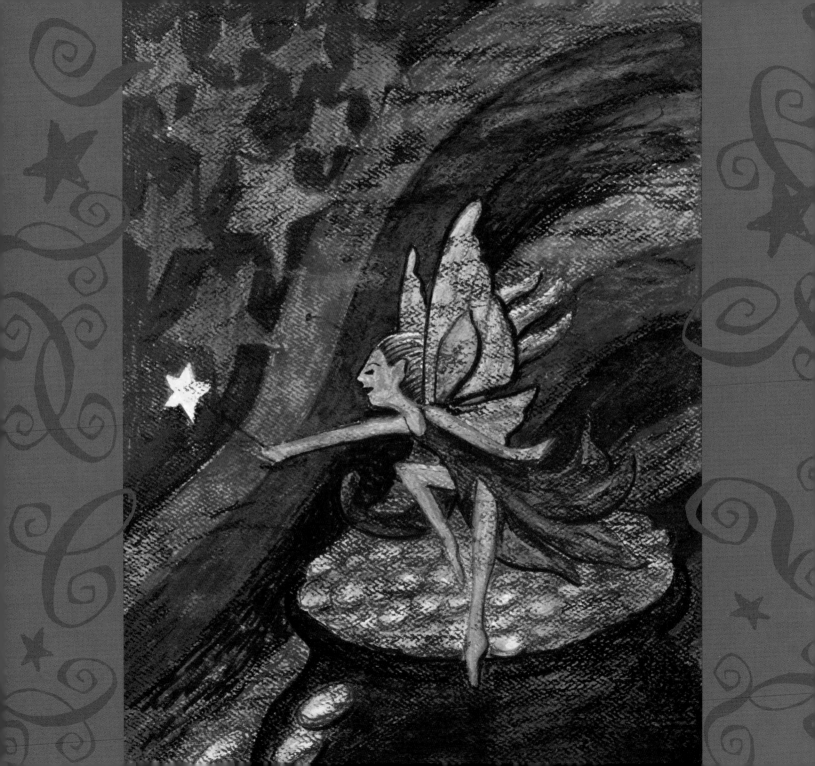

HOCUS POCUS FOCUS

To enlist the pixies and genies of success, and to conquer the dragons and trolls of frustration, you must focus on The Things That Matter. The wonder-working spells in this section will empower you to separate the ordinary from the important and to concentrate on the practices that create the biggest results.

You'll discover new wand-wielding magic for memory tricks and time wizardry. You'll learn to engage pixies, elves, genies and apprentice CLNC® wizards to create the office efficiencies that magically produce extra hours. You'll banish the Procrastination Gremlin and the Overwhelm Ogre from your magic carpet ride to the stars. You'll concentrate your sorcerer's energies for peak performance. You'll make time stand still and interruptions vanish.

You are in control of your magic show: behold your dazzling future—and hocus pocus focus.

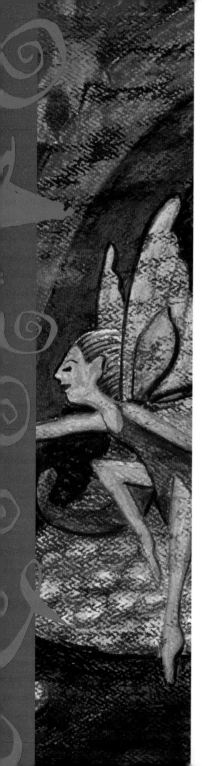

Don't Just Wish Upon a Star—Create One

Fairy godmothers and lamp genies are wonderful assistants, but when you want that dream to come true, a smart wizard doesn't wait for others to make it happen. Use this spell to open the gate to the yellow brick road that will take you wherever you want to go.

Start your magic spell with:

* A stack of interesting magazines
* A binder with a clear pocket on the front
* 3-hole paper
* Your CLNC® dream

Focus on the dream. The perfect time is during those magical twilight moments just before you fall asleep or just as you awake. If you had no limitations, what would your CLNC® dream be? See the dream in Technicolor detail. See it happening now.

Sit down with a stack of magazines and flip through pages until you feel a connection. It might be anything—a color, a beach, a tree, a brick walkway. Don't analyze it, just rip out the page, put it aside and keep going. Every time you feel a connection or see a fragment of an image that reminds you of that dream, tear it out.

Spread the pages all around you—on a table or the floor. Match compatible images, pages that just seem to go together. Choose the images that speak loudest and tear or cut them out. Paste them in a collage on a sheet of paper that slips into the clear front pocket of your dream binder. Add to your dream collage until it symbolizes artistically what you want in your life.

Imagine your dream in segments such as five or seven big events that lead to the final dream. Write those down. Now break down each segment into smaller steps. Think in terms of present-tense action verbs—call, write, make, do. If the steps are still too big, break them down further until you see a small step you can take right now—making a phone call, typing a list of supplies, creating a tickler file.

Program your mind toward success by verbally internalizing your plan. Do this daily, while putting on your clothes or booting up the computer.

Take that first step now.

The first 5 steps to realizing my CLNC® dream are

1. _____
2. _____
3. _____
4. _____
5. _____

> **Enchanter's Tip:** Identify the limiting step. Ghosties and ghoulies and long-legged beasties are never as frightening when we see them in the harsh light of day. Blocks that separate you from your dream become less overwhelming when you confront them head on. Smart wizards see stumbling blocks merely as stepping stones. How can you remove the block or go around it? Once you put that blockage behind you, the dream is yours. Embrace it. Tell your family about it. Tell other wizards. Build your enthusiasm for taking action daily.

A CODE FOR SUCCESS

- Action makes more fortunes than caution.

- If you aim at nothing you will hit nothing.

- Do not mistake activity for achievement.

- There are plenty of rules for success. None work unless you do.

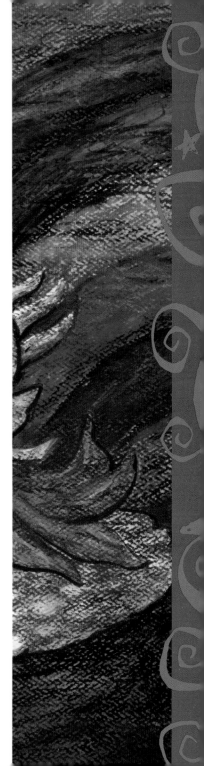

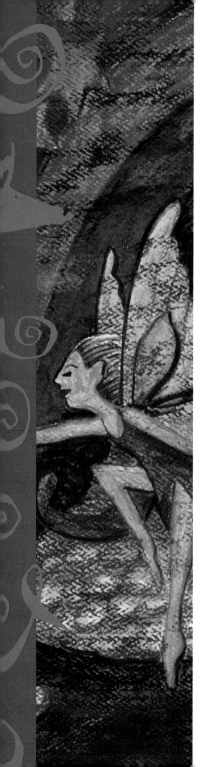

Focus on Your One Big Magic Trick

The pixies and elves clamor for attention, and it feels great to zip off an email that handles their dilemma. But what big thing did that email do for your business? Your day blossoms into dozens of niggling little tasks while the marketing plan is put off once again because it's "too big" to tackle in the amount of time left in your day. You'll never get to the Emerald City unless you start down that yellow brick road, one step at a time. Once you enjoy the accomplishment that comes from tackling something really big, you'll see that "over the rainbow" is not as far as it seems. Most importantly, you'll stay pumped all day from the glow of your accomplishments.

Prepare your time machine:

* Define the one big magic trick that will move your company forward
* Schedule a two-hour session during your peak performance time—ideally first thing in the morning, before the pixies and elves awaken

Start your spell by writing down five strategic imperatives, important but not urgent. Is it working on your information newsletter? Putting a dent in that in-depth report that's not due for three weeks? Interviewing two new prospects? Decide how each will impact your business. Start with the one that excites you the most.

Break your big thing into small, definable segments. Develop a project timeline and schedule a two-hour, power-hour session each day to complete it.

Delegate details that your team of pixies, elves and CLNC® subcontractors can handle.

Take action. Tackle the project and complete the first two-hour session. Avoid all interruptions such as phone calls and uninvited conversations.

Evaluate your efforts and start your next two-hour session.

Celebrate completing your one big magic trick.

My next big magic trick is

_____

_____

Pixie's Tip: Commitment to completing your one big thing is the most energizing elixir you can conjure. If you are struggling to manage interruptions, find a quiet spot away from your office to focus on your one big thing.

CREATE MAGIC WITH MESMERIZING FOCUS

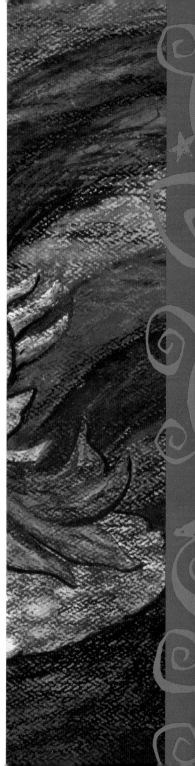

A crystal ball, a candle, a mantra—these magical devices focus your energy and thought into one powerful channel. By focusing all your concentration, you can move mountains. You can accomplish that report in record time or whip through research like a runaway broomstick. Use this spell for the self-enchantment that will improve your focus.

START YOUR ENCHANTMENT SPELL WITH:

* Ample clutter-free work space
* Appropriate lighting
* A comfortable desk chair
* Adequate office furniture and equipment with room to file all papers appropriately
* Silence, soft music or your favorite mantra (whichever works for you)

OPTIONAL ELIXIRS:

A User's Guide to the Brain
by John J. Ratey, M.D.

Tantric Heart, a CD by Shastro

Minimize distractions by working on one file or one conjuration at a time. Lay out only your current work on your desk.

Set a time limit to accomplish a specific spell or segment of a big project. Deadlines improve focus.

Simplify spells and incantations by using modern technology. Computers are artfully effective at word processing, time keeping, filing and tracking.

Improve concentration and attention to detail by keeping work in the office and out of the rest of the home.

Change locations to refocus on new projects.

Break up your day. If possible, don't stay on the same project all day. If you must complete a big project, break it into segments and refocus for each. Reward yourself with a short break after each 55-minute period of concentrated focus. The 55-minute period mirrors your brain's natural attention-sleep cycles.

Soothsayer's Advice: Concentration and attention to detail are essential to powerful spells, charms, elixirs and a high volume of excellent work product. Focus on the one thing that will generate the most dollars for you. Subcontract non-billable tasks. Gaze into the crystal ball and whisper, "hocus pocus focus," to zap yourself instantly back to CLNC® magician work.

SYMBOLS THAT ENCOURAGE FOCUS ON YOUR ONE BIG MAGIC TRICK

* A big $ dollar sign.
* A photo of the child you want to put through college.
* A dream vacation spot.
* A home, boat, auto or _____ you want to own.

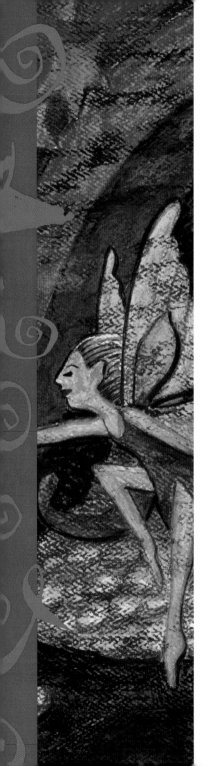

ADD TIME WIZARDRY TO YOUR MAGIC KIT

An efficient wizard can have elixirs to brew, spells to cast, a broomstick that needs tuning up before a scheduled moonlight ride, and still function with a clear head and a positive mental attitude. The secret is in seeing time as a valuable commodity.

ASSEMBLE YOUR CONJURER'S TOOLS:

* A clear and captivating overall vision
* A concise idea of the big goals you need to accomplish
* A list of specific "to do" items
* A calendar or electronic day planner
* A variety of colored highlighter markers

OPTIONAL ELIXIR:

***The Procrastinator's Handbook, Mastering the Art of Doing It Now* by Rita Emmett**

Develop a bewitching plan based on your vision. List the big goals you want to achieve in the following month, placing each project at the head of a column—marketing plan, tax projection, a book you want to read. Add a date to accomplish the goal. In the columns beneath, break down each project into segments, using as many as are practicable to complete by the deadline. Smaller projects always seem more manageable than huge ones.

On your monthly calendar, block out dates and times already committed, for example, client appointments, luncheons, kids' soccer games. Highlight business commitments in yellow, personal commitments in green and family commitments in orange. If using an electronic day planner, print out your monthly calendar.

* Schedule times to accomplish the big goals. Assign these to power hours. Highlight them in blue.
* Block out billable work periods to fulfill client projects and meet expected financial projections. Highlight these in pink.

On your weekly calendar, pencil in the scheduled commitments and billable work periods. Highlight these appropriately, then:

* Schedule time for yourself, highlighted in green.
* Use another color to mark items that don't fit into the categories above.

Study the monthly and weekly colors and notice the balance. If you see too much yellow, you could be overcommitting yourself for non-billable business engagements. If you see more blue, you might need to break down major projects into smaller segments. If you see more of any color, notice whether that is in balance with your overall vision.

On your daily calendar, make certain the appointments, major projects, billable work time and personal time are penciled in before scheduling daily housekeeping items like going to the supermarket or picking up the dry cleaning.

Prioritize and allot time increments for casting each spell and completing each task.

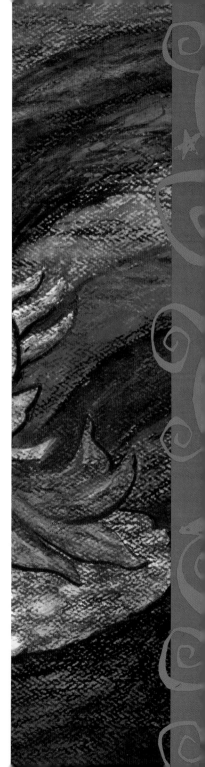

Wizard's Tip: Minutes of planning will save you hours of work. The planning exercise takes about 15 minutes a month, 10 minutes a week and 5 minutes a day. Make the time to plan and you'll magically get more done. When your sorcerer's spell book is so full that it allows no flexibility—and you see no white space on your calendar—you are overcommitted. Mark the tasks that can be delegated. Delegate them. Reprioritize. Eliminate. Reschedule. You are the CLNC® wizard of your own time.

Banish the Procrastination Gremlin and these 15 excuses that steal your time and your money

1. I work better under pressure.

2. I've got writer's block.

3. I need to do more research.

4. It might be important, but it's not urgent.

5. I keep forgetting.

6. It's boring.

7. I have too much on my plate right now.

8. I need to sleep on it.

9. I'll get to it, right after this TV program.

10. My astrology chart says not to.

11. It's such a lousy, rainy day.

12. It's such a beautiful, sunny day.

13. It's not due yet.

14. I'm too tired.

15. I feel too good now to make myself work.

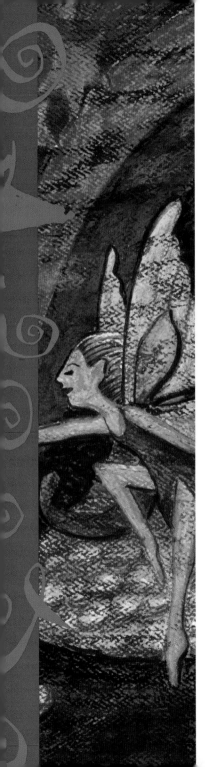

ᘿ Make Time Stand Still ᘿ

Every working wizard occasionally needs a few extra hours in a day. Time slides into cracks and vanishes. With this spell, you can stretch time to provide the extra hours you need.

Assemble your conjurer's tools:

✶ A clock
✶ A journal
✶ A pocket calendar or electronic day planner
✶ A housekeeper
✶ An assistant

Optional elixir:

Time-management books, such as *Getting Things Done: How to Achieve Stress-Free Productivity* by David Allen and *Time Management for the Creative Person* by Lee T. Silber

Journal your time for one week and identify time stealers. Recognize the time you spend:

• Watching TV
• Running errands
• Spending time on the Internet
• Chatting with fellow wizards
• Visiting the refrigerator and coffee pot

Work effectively by using your calendar to plan your day and to stay organized. Develop office systems to help you manage your day. Keep your office organized and clutter free. Set an egg timer for phone calls. Say "no" often, appreciating that what you say "no" to is just as important as what you say "yes" to.

Multitask:

• Tape your favorite news program to watch during routine activities such as exercising or sorting and filing.
• Walk while listening to CDs. You can even listen to your own recorded notes.
• Make routine phone calls while waiting in line or at the doctor's office.
• When on hold, use a headset to have both hands free for reading, working and sorting.

Take advantage of free delivery—office supplies, dry cleaning, groceries. Coordinate errands or hire someone to run errands. Hire a housekeeper and personal assistant.

Subcontract cases to another CLNC® consultant.

My biggest time stealer is

_____

Wizard's Wisdom: When despite all your multitasking and time-saving efforts you still need an extra witching hour, the magic that works best is your alarm clock. Set your alarm to wake you an hour earlier, or stay up an hour later (but not to watch TV).

Time is money

"Procrastination prevents success. Make today count. Use it or lose it. Do the worst first. Do it anyway! Life is leaking through your fingers. If it's worth doing, it's worth doing now. Winners don't wait."
—*Edwin C. Bliss*

ENjOY MORE TREATS
WITH THESE
MEMORY TRICKS

Perhaps you've already memorized a dozen uses for dragon's blood and the 105 distillations of common wolfbane, but if a dastardly wizard slips you a sip of forgetfulness serum, you'll make good use of this spell.

Start your incantation with:

✹ An appointment calendar with a "to-do" section or an electronic day planner and a pad of colorful Post-it® notes

Optional elixir:

A hand-held recorder

Don't rely on remembering something important. Write everything down *now*. Make lists or carry a small recorder for notes, and review them frequently.

Leave messages on your own voice mail and reminder notes on the steering wheel of your car, your bathroom mirror, refrigerator, phone—anywhere you know you can't help looking.

Maintain a detailed calendar—hard copy or electronic. Jot down phone numbers when you make appointments.

Before ending your workday, prepare all papers, files and supplies that you will need to take with you the following morning. Place them in your briefcase and place it inside the car.

Set an alarm or timer to remind you of specific tasks or phone calls you need to make.

> **Sorcerer's Secret:** We remember things when we focus on them, when we have passion for them and when they are loud, gaudy and obnoxious—whether we want to or not. Slow down a bit and allow yourself time to process new information. Simply using your brain keeps it strong. Exercise it by reading, doing puzzles, playing games or anything to keep the mind active. In your favorite cauldron, brew up the brain's preferred fuel—whole grains, fruits, vegetables and legumes.

Memory ticklers

Create a 12-month computer/PDA calendar with:

• Holidays, birthdays, anniversaries and recurring events.
• Due dates for BIG projects.
• Appointments and other commitments as they arise.

Set appropriate reminders: one week for big events, a day or two for appointments. Each week, scan your calendar for a mental update.

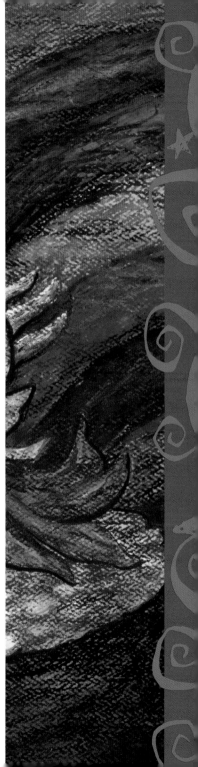

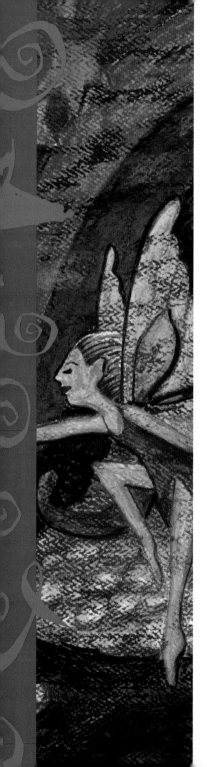

 # ZAP THE OVERWHELM OGRE

When the Wicked Witch of the West melted she was obviously in a state of overwhelm. Juggling all the necessary tasks in your new CLNC® practice can easily absorb all your time and energy. Add a family, a second job or any sort of social life, and you can feel as if there are not enough hours or elixirs in the day. Use this spell to zap overwhelm before that big splash of cold water melts you right down into a puddle.

Start your incantation with:

* A list of necessary tasks
* A daily, weekly and monthly schedule
* A support system of friends and colleagues
* CLNC® wizards
* Courage, patience, persistence and enthusiasm

Optional elixir:

Music or break-time activities that energize you

Prioritize your "to-do" lists monthly, weekly and daily. Look into the crystal ball for opportunities to subcontract or outsource. Delegate the least important tasks, or tasks that you don't feel quite ready to handle. Organize and schedule the projects you must handle yourself.

Take one thing at a time. Finish one objective before starting another. Tackle a small piece of a big project for that feeling of accomplishment, and check it off as you complete it.

Celebrate mini-accomplishments with a short break, a long, relaxing bath, an energizing drink or a treat that enchants your senses.

Learn to say "no" to distracting projects and activities that don't support your vision.

Call a supportive voice when you need suggestions, a sounding board for ideas, help in reevaluating your situation or just to indulge in a five-minute pity party. Then tackle the project with renewed enthusiasm.

Walk away or take a short broomstick ride. Get a fresh perspective. Remind yourself: you are only one wizard.

Leave work on time. Close the office door and banish work from your mind. The project will look clearer in the morning.

Wizard's Tip: Overwhelm is a temporary state of mind. You can beat it by focusing on one thing at a time. Mistrust either wild enthusiasm or deep dejection, both will hex you into losing your focus. Concentrate on the next thing to be done, then the next, ignoring the Overwhelm Ogre until he vanishes.

Axioms that work magic

Wisdom is knowing what to do next,
skill is knowing how, success is doing it.
You have to do a thing to learn how to do it.
It's the hard jobs that make us.

Delegate to CLNC® Subcontractors and Other Pixies and Elves

Pixies and elves can magically cut your work time in half and double your billable hours. Practice artful delegation and you can pull off the trick of being in two places at one time. Actively keep several pixies and elves busy, and you'll see the work magically accomplish itself, while your pot of gold overflows.

Activate your time warp with:

★ CLNC® subcontractors and expert witnesses

★ Other pixies and elves (family members, bookkeeper)

★ A list of strengths for each

★ A list of small potions to delegate that require minimal magic

★ A list of your weaknesses that pixies and elves can counteract

★ A list of tasks you enjoy too much

★ A list of non-business tasks to delegate

★ A follow-up system

Give yourself permission to hire CLNC® subcontractors, pixies and elves and to use the strengths and wisdom they bring to your business.

Begin your day by listing every task you can delegate. Delegate small spells and potions that the new CLNC® subs, pixies and elves can easily accomplish. Delegate to their strengths.

Delegate diplomatically and effectively by outlining clearly the expected results and the time allotted. Energize your helpers' enthusiasm for the tasks.

Schedule milestones and follow-up discussions to ensure the spell is working and will be completed on time.

Gradually delegate more important spells, tasks you tend to put off, tasks your CLNC® subs, pixies and elves are better qualified to do, or tasks you enjoy but cannot bill at the highest rate.

Meet with your CLNC® subs, pixies and elves regularly to brainstorm ideas and discuss results.

Sorcerer's Tip: Avoid micromanaging. Let your CLNC® subs, pixies and elves work their own magic to achieve amazing results. Celebrate accomplishments. Lavish them with praise and give criticism sparingly and concisely.

Tiny pixies and elves make excellent apprentices
Delegate creatively to your children and grandchildren

Resources for locating excellent CLNC® subcontractors
NACLNC® Conference and the NACLNC® Online Directory

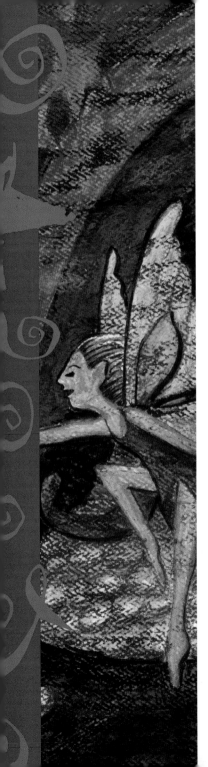

Banish Home Office Interruptions

Y ou've carefully measured the eel's eyes and toad's toes, stirred in a teaspoon of unicorn horn, and the cauldron has come to just the right bubble. You start the incantation and the phone rings. *Drat!* Do you allow an unscheduled caller to ruin your concentration? Not if you first empower this spell.

Assemble your sorcerer's tools:

* Voice mail
* Preschool, day care, a babysitter or other charms to handle the kids

Optional elixir:

An administrative assistant—possibly a family member

Designate an interruption-free work period and establish an isolated place to work—away from distractions. Make that space inviolate. During this time, allow voice mail to take the phone calls, put a "do not disturb" sign on your door and close it. Ignore the knocking, even if you hear a dragon roaring outside.

Set priorities for the day's conjurations and expected times for project completions.

Schedule a time to return phone calls and answer email. Stand when talking on the phone. Set an egg timer, and have a script memorized for politely ending a call.

Consider doing intensive projects off-site at a local library, a church or at home if your professional office is outside the home.

Tell all vendors to call during specified hours. Let friends and family know when your wizard's workday begins and ends. Plan inclusive activities during your off-time hours, so that friends and family don't feel abandoned.

My official workday begins at

_____ and ends at _____

> **Wizard's Tip:** You can be the master of time or the slave of interruptions. The choice is yours. Don't give in to home office distractions—TV, household chores, friendly chats. They will eat away time designated for your business—and time is money. Schedule such activities during your break time or at the end of the workday—after the spells are all cast, the elixirs have been bottled and the cauldron is off the fire.

Manage an uninvited visitor

If, despite your resolve, an uninvited visitor gets inside your office door, don't offer a chair. Stand up and remain standing. Set a time limit for this distraction and have a script memorized (*"I'm going to get back to work now"*) to politely ask the person to leave.

If the interruption is necessary but delaying it would be helpful, announce the times you are accessible. Say, "I would like to discuss this with you. Can we do it at 4:00pm?"

Control Your CLNC® Magic Show

Every CLNC® wizard needs a measure of circumspection and prudence in setting the attorney-client relationship boundaries. You are not a paralegal. While your sorcerer's skills might overlap, you have distinctive experience and expertise that a paralegal does not have. Although you certainly want to maintain a friendly business relationship, you are not a bosom buddy or potential date. The perfect measure of mutual peer respect and professional courtesy makes the most alchemistic working relationship.

Start your magic spell with:

* Attorneys you want as clients
* Your stated CLNC® services
* Your stated fees and billing cycle

Educate your attorney-clients, beginning with the first job, to respect your expertise. Show that you're good at what you do by delivering excellent work product. Demonstrate your attention to detail. Give a little extra on those early assignments to expose the client to additional CLNC® services not yet requested. Ask if the attorney uses MDs, then explain how your expertise differs and better complements what the attorney needs—at a better rate.

Set consultation limits. Learn to say "no" to requests that take you outside of your CLNC® role. If asked to do legal research, for example, politely explain how your CLNC® skills fill a totally different purpose from a paralegal's. Educate the attorney about the 30 CLNC® services you can provide.

Set rush limits. Highlight the added benefits the attorney might have received if you had been given the case earlier. Ask regular clients, "What do you have coming in right now?" If an attorney persists in calling you at the last minute, politely explain that you cannot do your best work without adequate time. For repeat offenders, decide whether the account is worth the aggravation. If not, consider charging a rush fee. "I have other cases ahead of this, but if you're willing to pay a rush fee I can rearrange my schedule."

Set ethical limits. Do not accept unethical behavior such as padding your charges so the attorney can collect higher fees. Do not accept contingency-based fees. If a suggestion feels unethical to you, contact the State Bar.

Set pay limits. You deserve to be paid on time. If an attorney is persistently slow in paying your invoice, start collecting 100% of the projected budget up front.

Set personal limits. Keep meetings professional, whether in the office or out. Dress and act appropriately to maintain a professional distance, and expect the client to do likewise.

> **Sorcerer's Tip:** If a client repeatedly oversteps the boundaries, don't keep going back for more. Wave your magic wand, say the magic words and make the troll disappear, or at least raise your fee high enough to cover for the offensive troll odors.

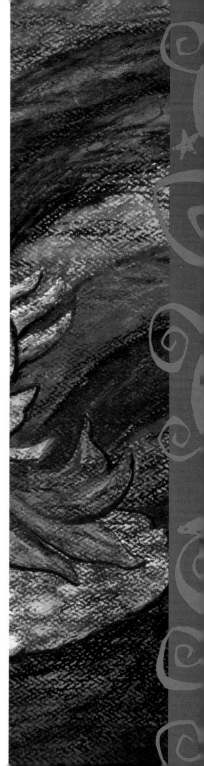

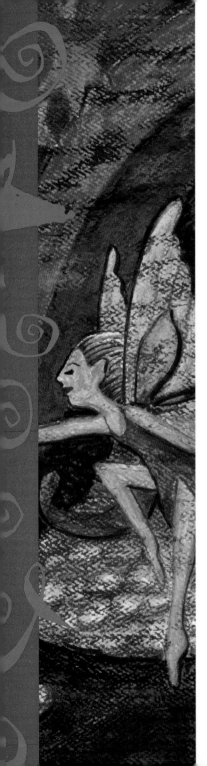

Manage Your Email Tollbooth Effectively

Residing in your computer is a phantom tollbooth marking the entrance to the Internet expressway and your online mailbox. The tollbooth has a magical window that provides instant communication with clients and access to research material. Used effectively, the window will save you hours of time over other forms of communication and research. But get bewitched by the tollbooth and you could be stuck there forever, wandering with Milo and Tock in The Lands Beyond.

Start your enchantment with:

* A computer, modem and monitor
* Internet access
* A clock
* A sorting hat

Create an email signature byline with your company name, contact information and a brief benefit-laden description of your CLNC® services. Use a professional-sounding email address and update your address book regularly.

Set specific times to respond to email during nonpeak work hours such as first thing in the morning, after lunch or at the end of the day. Turn off the chime and flashing icon.

Put on your sorting hat before you sit down to open your email. Delete unwanted mail liberally and quickly. Prioritize all emails that need immediate response and plan a time to respond to the others.

Create email folders for clinical topics, experts, prospects and marketing potions.

Install spam filtering software to divert spam to its own folder.

Print out important or sensitive emails as backup for your email folders.

Send less to receive less.

Compose your outgoing email messages as carefully as you would write a formal letter. Take the time to think about what you're saying. Write long or important emails in a word processing program first, then print out, proof, copy and paste. This can save you hours of materializing witchery if your email crashes.

To avoid forgetting the attachments, click "attach" first, *then* compose the email.

Set your email program to automatically spell check, but don't rely on it completely—proofread, proofread, proofread.

Take Sunday and vacations off from email.

Merlin's Tip: An email to a client represents you and your company as surely as does your business card or brochure. Without being too "cute," create emails that get the attention they deserve. Make the subject line relevant, compelling and descriptive. Use all your bewitchments to make the subject line tell a story that entices reading.

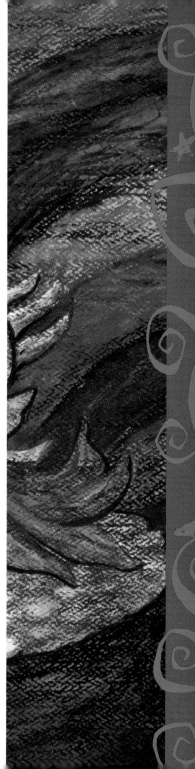

Moonlight to Illuminate Your Path to the Ball

As you accelerate from part-time to full-time CLNC® wizard, you'll be wearing two different hats. Like Cinderella, you'll continue sweeping the cinders as necessary so that you can dance later at the ball. Use this spell to avoid overwhelm and accomplish your goal of becoming a full-time Certified Legal Nurse Consultant^CM.

Assemble your conjurer's tools:

✷ A day planner (preferably electronic) or calendar

✷ A designated schedule for both jobs

Optional elixir:

***The Treasury of Quotes* by Jim Rohn and E. James Rohn**

Cast the runes and plan ahead to make your CLNC® business full time.

• Be open to working alternative schedules, such as three 12-hour weekend days, to free you up during the week.

• Project dates when you can financially phase down clinical practice to two days a week and phase up CLNC® projects to four days a week.

• Then project a date when you will take the next phase-down step in clinical practice to reach your full-time CLNC® goal.

Compartmentalize each job and conjure a magical cocoon to put yourself totally into the activity at hand. As philosophical wizard E. James Rohn says, "Wherever you are, be there."

Prepare mentally to work long hours. Exercise and take your vitamins for energy. Pace yourself and always keep your long-term goal in mind.

When you feel stressed, activate your memory spell and recall why you are doing this.

I will be a full-time CLNC® wizard by

> **Shaman's Secret:** You have the courage, enthusiasm, patience and persistence to undertake a journey that many would only dream of. Dreams can work magic, but only if you diligently cast the spells, work the charms and focus your energy on achieving your goal. The few who do are the envy of the many who only watch.

America is unique because it offers an economic ladder to climb.
And here's what's exciting: it is the bottom of the ladder that's crowded, not the top.
In America, everything you need to succeed is within reach.

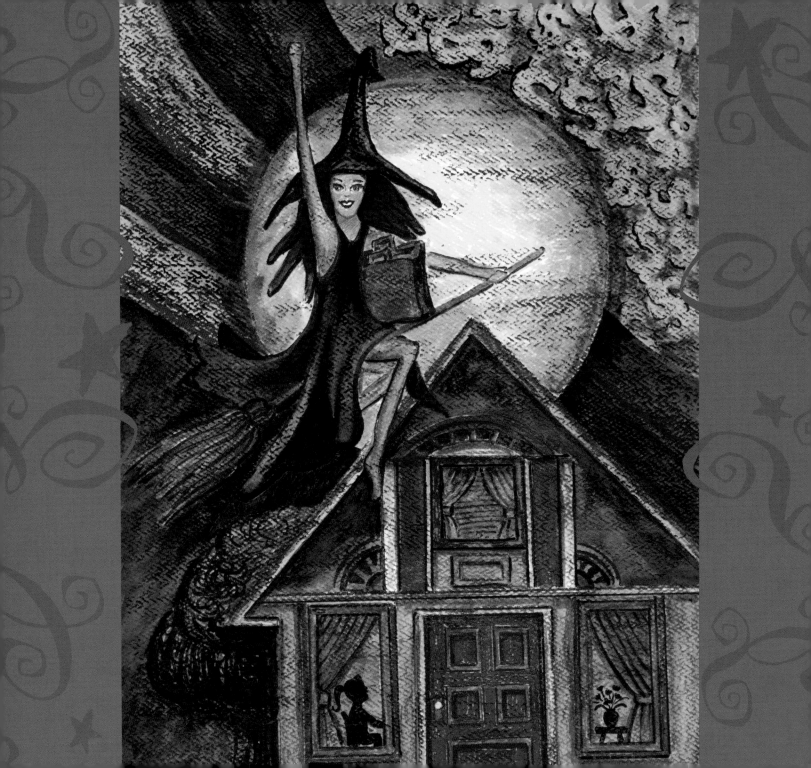

Keep Your Wizard's Workshop Lustrous

A place for everything and everything in its place. In an orderly world creativity and productivity flourish. Your sorcerer's hat hangs solidly on the hat tree. Your wand lies at hand. Your crystal ball awaits, polished and powerful. Eels' eyes, crows' claws and toads' toes, all in their proper jars, stand ready for the most delicately potent elixirs. Confusing the containers could prove disastrous.

Even when all the world is in chaos, a clever wizard commands an oasis of calm in her splendidly tricked-out workshop.

Use the hexes and potions that follow to demystify technology, create office efficiencies and assemble the complete, organized and lustrous wizard's workshop to support your CLNC® vision. Then revel in the power of order.

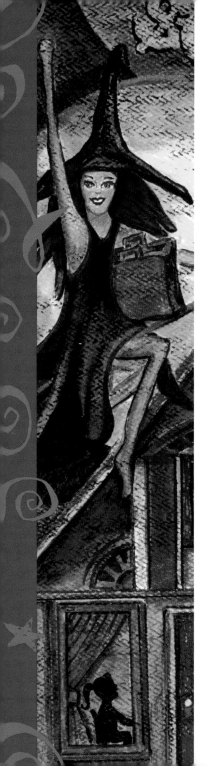

Demystify Technology

The wizard's computer is a magic wand that transfigures ideas into neatly printed reports, collapses reams of hard-copy files into an invisible micro-space until you need them and provides a fascinating window to your universe. Don't be afraid. If you press the wrong key, the computer won't blow up or turn you into a frog.

Start your incantation with:

* An allotted time to play and practice
* Program tutorials
* A list of local computer classes

Optional elixir:

A step-by-step "Dummies" book

Decide which type of learner you are. Do you enjoy reading and discovering on your own? Or do you prefer the personal touch—a buddy wizard to walk you through? Or perhaps you would feel more comfortable learning in a classroom from a master wizard. Whichever you choose, the basics are easier than you might think.

Take the time to go through tutorials. Read directions and use the "help" function. When lost, click the helpful icons and cues to guide you and always be sure to read the screen.

Laugh at and learn from your mistakes. It's only a computer—designed by engineers and therefore not necessarily logical.

Read directions. Every program has important information available on the screen, in a manual or in a "help" file.

Remember to save your work frequently. Every 5 or 10 minutes is not too often.

Learn keyboard shortcuts. These can save you loads of time.

Wizard's Tip: You're smart enough to learn computer skills, but perhaps that's not where you want to use your valuable time. In that case, hire a tech wizard to do it for you. Perhaps you have a family member who is a computer whiz or you know a local college student who needs part-time work. Most young people grew up using computers and can accomplish in minutes what might take a nontechnical sorcerer tedious hours to master. I built my company with no technology expertise. Decades later little has changed in that regard. I merely conjure up a tech-elf whenever I need one.

A sample spell that works magic

When you find yourself frustrated with learning your way around a computer, remember what Mark Twain called the greatest of all inventors: accident.

ORGANIZE YOUR WIZARD'S WORKSHOP

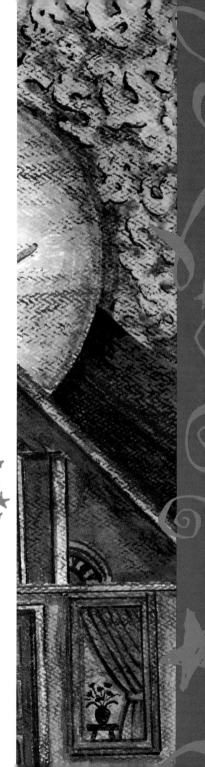

Who doesn't wish for a crystal ball to help find the file you misplaced? Or a Ouija board to tell you the name of that prospect you intended to call? Or a friendly lamp genie, who with one *whish!* will zap a messy office into sparkling organization? An orderly office saves you hours each week in wasted time, and getting there is as easy as *open sesame* when you invoke this daily spell.

SUMMON YOUR OFFICE GENIE WITH:

* Adequate work space with a place for everything
* Appropriate equipment and supplies

OPTIONAL ELIXIR:

Rented off-site storage for old files that cannot be destroyed

The genie's secret for organization is to *start* organized. Create a filing system for all records, research and case materials. Color-coding will make everything easier to identify. To eliminate stacks, file or destroy every piece of paper that crosses your desk. Manage phone messages and emails daily. Keep your attorney-client list, contact list and subcontractor list current. Make good use of the trash can, shredder and "delete" button.

Define creativity pockets—areas that remain clutter free at all times—for reading, writing and brainstorming activities.

Prepare for emergencies by having a written back-up plan for systems failure—computer, fax machine, printer and telephone.

Designate a cut-off time each day to stop working and reorganize your work space. Organize your day each morning. Assign one day each month for complete housekeeping—finish early and take the rest of the day off.

> **Aladdin's Advice:** You use less than 10% of the material you file. Purge, archive or destroy records on a regular basis. Zap that pile of mail into the trash can and those extra copies into the shredder. You'll have 90% more space and more time to allocate to billable hours.

An ideal office

Desk, ergonomically designed chair, file cabinet, bookshelves, telephone with dedicated phone lines, computer with contact management software, good work light, Internet connection, Physician's Desk Reference (PDR), organizing tray for miscellaneous items, adequate supplies, trash can, shredder and a door that closes.

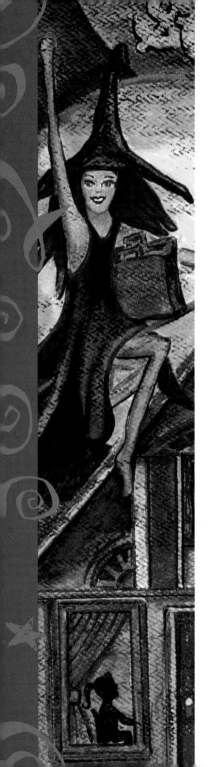

Design Your Wizard's Workshop for Efficiency

The efficient wizard keeps her crystal ball polished, her thinking cap handy and her broomstick tuned up. Office efficiencies eliminate wasted time, which creates extra hours for billable time. Use this spell to sharpen your office operations.

Start your magic spell with:

* An energy-efficient office layout
* Essential office furniture and equipment
* A wickedly good filing system

Optional elixir:

Organization books, such as *Taming the Paper Tiger at Work* and *Taming the Paper Tiger at Home*, both by Barbara Hemphill

Computerize—and learn to use software shortcuts. Invest time in mastering all the word processing, bookkeeping, filing, sorting, printing and mailing features of your computer.

Create systems for day-to-day operations. Avoid stacks and piles. Keep the work space clear and the work flowing.

Create templates for reports, invoicing, agreements, incantations and contracts. Don't reinvent the wheel. Reuse components of letters, reports, articles and speeches.

Program the speed dial function on your phone and fax.

Outsource filing, sorting and other tasks to allow efficient use of your most productive hours.

Have a back-up plan for anticipated equipment failure. Downtime is lost time, and time is money. Develop a simple method for maintaining an inventory of office supplies and bewitching tools.

> **Wizard's Tip:** An organized, clutter-free work space—with bewitching tools in their proper place, conjuring equipment primed and ready, an invigorating atmosphere and a clock in clear view—invites you to get busy. Jumbled papers and ill-kept equipment encourages procrastination and inefficiency. You waste the first minutes getting organized and locating the materials you need, which is a mental and psychological roadblock to efficiently managing your work. Instead, tidy up. Tuck away files, charms, crystals and cauldrons. Leave your office organized each evening. Return the next morning to a mystically energizing and efficient environment.

A 3 D incantation

Avoid setting things aside to be done later. Use the 3 Ds method—Do it, Ditch it or Delegate it. Tie up loose ends before putting away each project. Reorganize your desk before you take out the next project. Schedule tomorrow before you retire today.

ASSEMBLE THE COMPLETE WIZARD'S WORKSHOP

Bell, book and incredible candles—a wizard is only as good as her tools. The magic of doing business requires certain essentials at start-up. Other items can be acquired as your business progresses and your profits mount. A smart sorcerer knows the difference between immediately essential equipment and a wish list of wickedly desirable but secondary conveniences. When in doubt, consult this oracle.

THE ESSENTIAL CLNC® WIZARD'S WORKSHOP:

* Crystal ball, cauldron and magic wand
* An ergonomic chair
* Adequate work space in your castle
* Professional business cards and stationery
* Postal mailbox address
* Computer, printer and word processing software (e.g., Word)
* Fax machine access
* Power surge protector
* High-speed Internet access and email
* Basic reference materials
* Basic supplies including computer paper, legal pads, postage stamps, pens, highlighters, paper clips, a stapler, file folders, in/out baskets, color-coded legal files
* A filing cabinet
* Cell phone

THE CLNC® WIZARD'S WORKSHOP LUXURY ITEMS:

* First-class office furniture, including a spacious desk and credenza
* Dedicated business lines for equipment
* Scanner
* Copy machine
* Additional printer, preferably color
* Back-up system for all equipment
* Specialized software for bookkeeping, contact management, research
* Elegant business stationery, personalized note cards, Post-it® notes with your company name, address and contact information
* Medical reference library
* Electronic day planner
* Electronic business cards, CD or DVD explaining your services

Soothsayer's Secret: Allow demand to dictate acquisition. Invest in your dream, but if you forestall purchasing desirable yet nonessential office equipment, you'll have more opportunities to enjoy your wizard's rewards. Take that rapturous long-awaited trip to the office supply store to celebrate your successes.

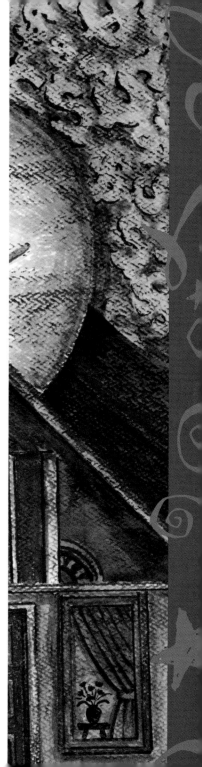

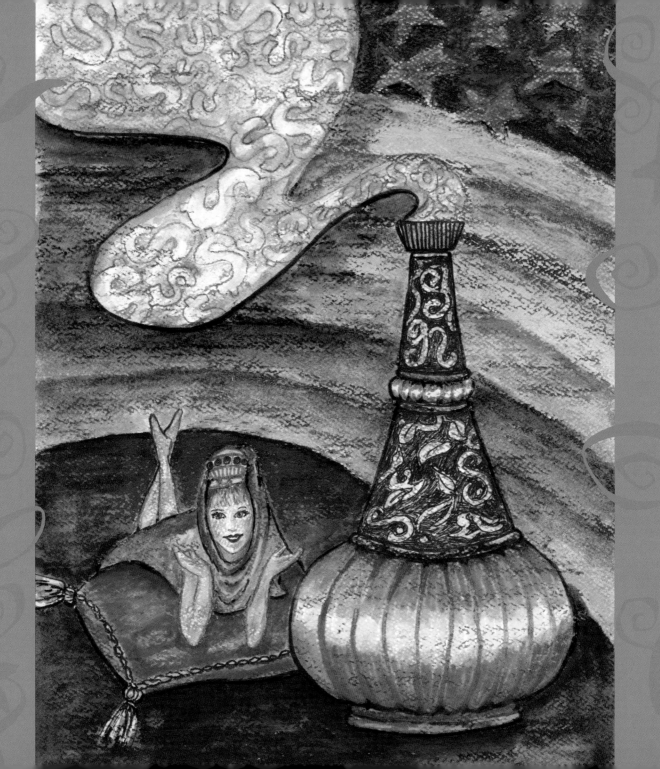

Unleash Your Genie to Tackle Unique Business Challenges

Rub the magic lamp and your genie emerges with the extraordinary tricks, techniques and talent you'll need when unique business challenges occur. With a twitch of your nose you'll vanquish unreasonable clients. In the blink of an eye you'll steer your magic carpet nimbly around conflicts of interest. With three clicks of your ruby slippers you'll successfully relocate your business from Kansas to Oz and gain new clients in the process.

This is the time to roll up the sleeves of your conjuring robe and studiously practice your craft. While everyday magic will whisk you through routine business days, when the biggest, ugliest, meanest dragons roar, you'll use the following spells to unleash your genie and put out the fires.

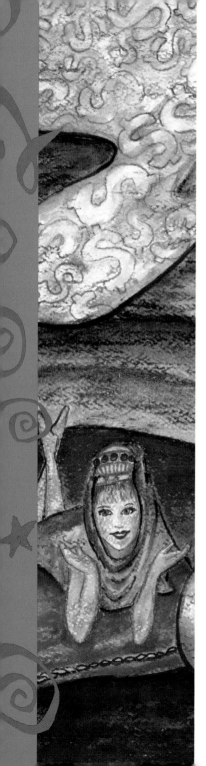

Steer Your Magic Carpet around Conflicts of Interest

A desirable high-dollar case can work like a Pied Piper's flute, luring you into dangerous situations. When a legal nurse consultant cannot be objective, or will be perceived as not being objective, the work product—no matter how dazzling—might ultimately damage the case. Use this elixir to banish the Pied Piper's music and perform your magic with integrity.

Start your magic elixir with:

★ A wizardly quantity of ethics

★ A cup of common sense

★ A dash of courage

★ A sprinkle of tact

Identify the conflict. Do you:

• Feel you cannot be objective because you know the defendants, demons, trolls, experts or other players?

• Work in the institution being sued?

• Work in a clinic or hospital or the corporation affiliated with the defendant-institution?

If you clearly have a conflict, tell the attorney why you cannot work on the case.

If the conflict is questionable, discuss it with the attorney and seek his opinion regarding whether you should work the case.

> **Soothsayer's Advice for Expert Witnesses:** Ignoring the Piper's music is not always easy. When you believe you can be objective and you know you can do an excellent job as an expert witness, you might feel drawn into going forward. However, the perception of conflict is enough for the court to take wicked exception, which will discredit you, your testimony and the attorney. This is an excellent time to step aside and cast the runes for another able CLNC® consultant.

Tame the Personal Challenge Demon

What image comes to mind when you think of Cinderella—beautiful ball gown, glass slipper, handsome prince? Most of us forget that before the fairy godmother showed up, Cinderella had lost everything. Her widowed father married a harridan with two mean daughters, and at her father's death, Cinderella became her stepmother's slave. What a crisis! Divorce, death, illness, menopause and physical challenges can create stumbling blocks for any business, but this potion can set you firmly back on your path.

Create your magic potion with:

✳ A back-up system complete with a network of CLNC® subcontractors

✳ An emotional support system of friends and family to whom you can talk

✳ Your *I Am a Successful CLNC® Success Journal*

✳ A magical health regimen—diet, exercise, a good night's rest

✳ Professional help as needed

Optional elixir:

Inspirational books, such as *Final Gifts* by Maggie Callanan and Patricia Kelley

Step back to see the whole picture. What's the magnitude of this challenge? What are the specific obstacles and hurdles to overcome? Develop a mind-set that nothing can stop you. Focus on what you can and must do rather than on the difficulties or limitations. Give yourself permission to deal with the challenge.

Reset your priorities to deal with the crisis until resolved. Delegate business matters that another wizard can handle, then reprioritize projects that need your personal attention. A crisis takes priority, but mundane tasks can provide mental and emotional relief.

Call on your trusted CLNC® subcontractors and assure key clients that their needs will continue to be satisfied.

Don't share your crises with clients unless you absolutely must. Then do so without emotion.

Maintain your sense of humor and your physical and spiritual balance during the crisis. Banish negative thoughts. Read inspirational texts and write in your sorcerer's *CLNC® Success Journal* to help clear your mind. When your spirits need a quick boost, treat yourself to a captivating new hair style or a bewitching movie.

View all obstacles and crises as simply challenges. You can lower your anxiety by viewing a situation as less extreme than you originally imagined. An insurmountable mountain is no problem for a wickedly fast Nimbus 2000 broomstick.

> **Wizard's Tip:** In a herd of elephants, when one falls, the others pick him up. Surround yourself with your own family of elephants—friends and family you love and who love you. Focus on the positive elements in your life. Breathe deeply, forget those fireplace cinders that need sweeping and think about your compelling reasons for maintaining your business during this trying period.

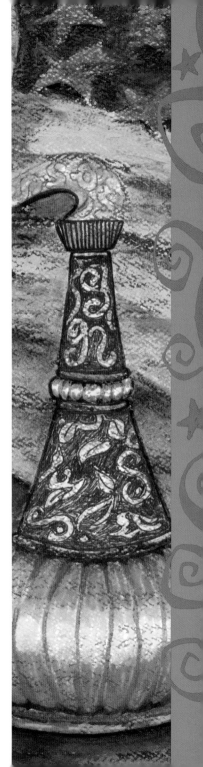

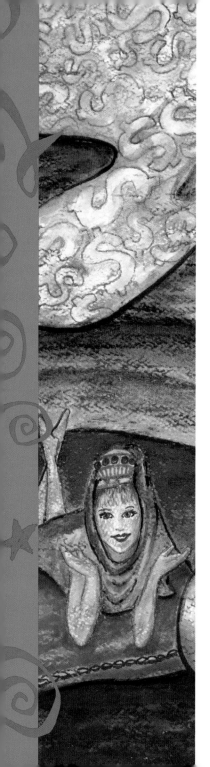

 # CHARM DIFFICULT ATTORNEYS

A charm is powerful magic, and every good wizard is a charms master. Charm is an important tool when you're faced with an attorney-client who makes your job difficult. However, if Beauty had not seen past the Beast's surly attitude and nasty temper, they would never have become friends. If the client relationship is worth saving, this magical spell will make it happen.

START YOUR CHARMING SPELL WITH:

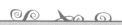

* A win-win attitude
* An open mind to the possibility of change

OPTIONAL ELIXIR:

***Mars and Venus in the Workplace* by John Gray**

Identify the problematic issue and focus the conversation on resolving that issue. If your attorney-client draws you in another direction, acknowledge the drift with a comment such as, "that may be relevant, but let's save it for later," and firmly return to the key issue.

Hear the attorney out before commenting. Listen. Acknowledge that you are listening by mirroring gestures and repeating key words.

Set limits. Do not allow rudeness, crudeness or disrespect. If a client speaks brusquely, ignore the tone and volume, and move the conversation to a more professional and friendly spirit. The attorney will automatically mirror the change. This enchantment is powerful.

Don't be intimidated. Remember, you are the nursing wizard. The attorney needs your services. If you cannot work together, find a CLNC® sub to match the attorney's personality—and *bibbity, bobbity, boo!*—you're out of the conflict without losing the business.

> **Soothsayer's Tip:** One of the most powerful charms at your disposal is the wizard's way of congeniality. If the client is important to you, make a comment such as, "I see this is not working. What do you want to realize as an outcome?" If fair and reasonable, then do what the attorney has asked. Magic is not always complicated.

PROFILE OF AN IDEAL ATTORNEY-CLIENT

* Appreciates your services as a CLNC® consultant.
* Is professional, respectful, ethical and fun to work with.
* Is passionate and caring about cases.
* Is an excellent communicator.
* Calls you on a timely basis.
* Trusts your judgment.
* Empowers you to do what's needed.
* Values you as a member of the team.
* Listens to your opinions.
* Pays on time.
* Enjoys paying what you're worth.
* Refers your services to other attorneys.

Make Serpents and Other Difficult Clients Disappear

Every good magician has a vanishing act. And what better time to use it than when a client becomes so difficult that your yellow brick road leads to a towering headache? When you feel like waving your wand and dropping a house on your client's head, here's a potion that's just the trick.

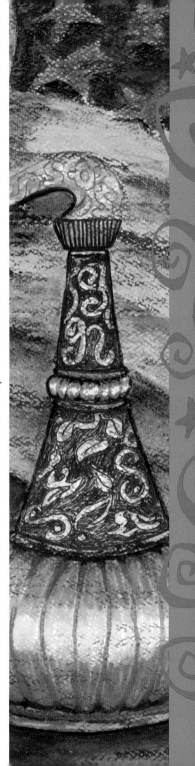

Meditate on your client's wicked ways:

* Calls at the 11th hour
* Sets arbitrary deadlines
* Demands unreasonable results
* Skimps on the budget
* Lacks ethics and integrity
* Consistently pays late
* Is inconsiderate, condescending or unappreciative
* Keeps you up at night

Mix a quick, offensive repellent:

Double your fees and require 100% retainer up front.

Soothsayer's Advice: If the attorney-client swallows the potion and fails to vanish, consider one wizard's sage decision, "For that amount of money, he's not so difficult." If the client survives the potion and is too wicked at any amount of money, use a vanishing trick on yourself and simply become too busy to accept the client's work.

A devilishly delightful elixir

Draw a bath. Add six drops of orange oil or two lemons sliced into wheels.
Rub your skin lightly all over with a dry loofah, a dry coarse sponge or a natural-bristle brush.
Relax and soak for 15 minutes while sipping your favorite beverage.

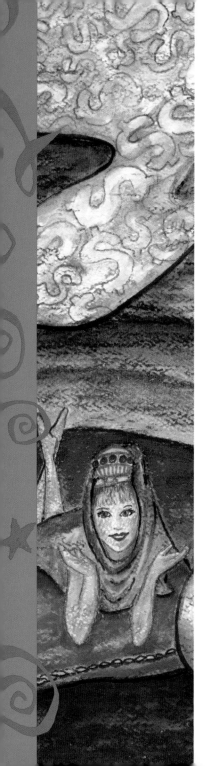

Simplify Your Magic Carpet Travel

Leaving your castle on a business trip can be exciting or traumatic, depending on your preparation. Before you ride off on your magic carpet, take the time to apply these travel incantations. You'll have fewer hexes, jinxes and hassles and arrive ready for business.

Start your enchanting ride with:

✳ Rolling luggage
✳ An organizer for the photo ID you'll frequently need to show
✳ Comfortable clothes that don't wrinkle

Plan your clothing needs before you pack by doing what fashion wizards do to prepare for photo shoots—lay all the pieces of each outfit together on your bed and coordinate everything, including accessories. Tuck a packing list in your suitcase for next time.

Pack light. Take a mix-and-match separates wardrobe in a single color scheme. This will eliminate extra shoes and accessories.

Take an expense log to track your business travel expenses, and a large envelope to save receipts.

If driving, have a good map and directions. Leave all travel items in the trunk.

If flying, travel in the early morning. You will encounter fewer delays. Allow time to make connecting flights, and book direct flights when possible. Ask to be seated away from the galley, bathroom or bulkhead, so that you can work or relax. Sign up for a frequent flyer card.

• Make sure to bring necessary business documents and plenty of work to do in your carry-on bag. This eases the stress of delays.

• Don't put all your money in the same bag. Put a little in your carry-on and a little in your wallet. Empty your wallet of nonessential information.

• Be safe—don't put your name and address where it's visible.

• Never check your laptop computer. Use a bag with a side zipper so that you can slide the laptop out at the inspection counter. Take an extra charged battery or an airplane power adapter.

Arrive early and freshen up in the restroom before your meeting.

Sage's Advice: Ask a neighbor or family member to watch over your CLNC® kingdom. Have two copies of valuable documents, such as driver's license and credit cards. Leave one with a trusted elf and carry one with you. Store toiletries in a sealed bag to prevent leakage. Pack a luggage tag inside your luggage. Place a bright handle wrap on your luggage.

Sprinkle your magic carpet travel with pixie dust

Carry on anything you cannot do without. Place your bags on the conveyor belt right when you are ready to walk through the scanner. Always keep some reading handy. Carry a bottle of water—you will need a drink before your magic carpet lands safely.

Relocate Your Business from Kansas to Oz with 3 Clicks

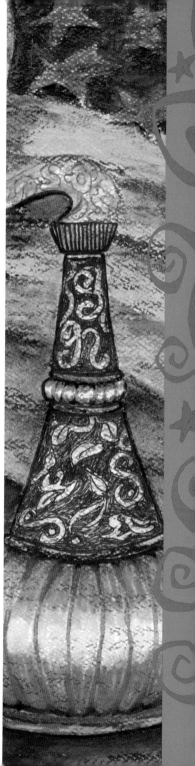

Grab your belongings, click your ruby-slippered heels together three times and *zap!* you and your business appear in a bustling new city and state. Can it be that easy? With this spell, you'll smooth out all the bumps.

Start your relocation spell with:

* A commitment to relocate
* A new promotional package that includes your new contact information
* A new state RN license
* Yellow Pages for your new city
* A contact at the state bar, plaintiff/defense bar and county or city bar
* A list of upcoming legal conferences
* Local legal journals
* Your information newsletter
* A list of CLNC® wizards in your new city

Long before your move date, research and establish contacts in the new location. At the same time, cement your current attorney-client relationships. Don't allow clients to feel abandoned. Make arrangements for them to find you easily (fax, FedEx, email, U.S. mail).

Send a move announcement to attorney-clients, vendors, fellow CLNC® wizards, your mentors at Vickie Milazzo Institute and others, then print the announcement in your newsletter and mail it to attorneys and other contacts in the new city.

Ask existing attorney-clients and everyone you know for names of attorneys in your new location.

Write an article for a legal journal in your new state.

Arrange to exhibit at the next legal conference in your new state.

Attend local chamber and business functions and connect with your new community. Offer to speak at law offices, insurance companies, business breakfasts, luncheons and other gatherings.

During the move, maintain the security of active files.

Soothsayer's Advice: Don your most impressive wizard's cloak and spend a day visiting with key attorneys in the new community. Let them know the skills and experience that just magically arrived to help them. Drop names of firms with which you've worked. By establishing yourself before the move, you create a warm welcome. When anticipation magically replaces anxiety, your trek down the yellow brick road will be enchantingly rewarding. Plus you get a whole new office in your new castle.

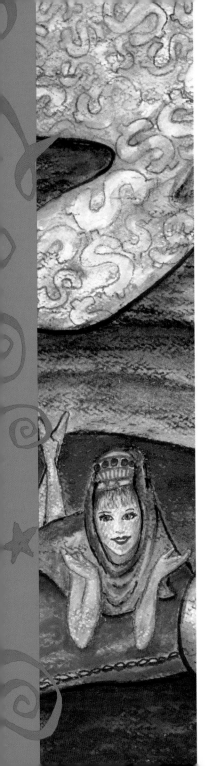

It's Not Such a Small, Small World Working in a Rural Environment

Wizards often find themselves most comfortable outside the bustle and hassle of urban activity. For the CLNC® wizard, however, this poses a dilemma—the number of attorneys within the range of your incantation might not support a burgeoning business. You'll need this very specific spell to reach out and enchant a wider community. They'll forget you're from Kansas and think you're from Oz.

Start your rural environment spell with:

* A conviction to succeed
* The names of the three nearest urban locations
* A list of business groups
* A computer and printer
* A scanner and/or copier
* A toll-free number
* Internet access
* A wickedly fast broomstick
* Wasp and hornet spray

Anticipate the environmental limitations of your area and make a plan to overcome them. Secure adequate communication. This is essential, because your clients need to feel that you're as close as a phone call. Learn to use email effectively. Establish personal contact with delivery sources—FedEx, UPS, U.S. mail—and make friends with the local attendant or driver.

Be willing to travel. Your initial meeting with attorneys should be face-to-face. Never let a prospect or client visit your rural location before you have met them in their business office.

Join a business group in your target city that meets once a month. This will ensure that you visit your market at least monthly. Schedule prospect and client meetings on that same day.

Allow time for the unexpected. Be ready to combat wasps and hornets. Never let your rural location compromise your client relationships.

My next visit to my target city

is _____ (DATE)

> **Wizard's Tip:** Modern technology impressively widens a wizard's scope of influence. Make use of your telephone and email and otherwise keep in touch daily to enchant your prospects, clients and business associates.

Being from a small rural community and not knowing any attorneys personally could have stopped me from pursuing my dream. But I knew there was more out there if I would "dare to dream!"

One of the things I love about this business and being a Certified Legal Nurse Consultant[CM] is that the harder I work, the more I get rewarded. That's not usually the case in hospitals, which is frustrating. When I first began, even before I went full time, I replaced my annual nurse's salary within six months. And once I left the hospital, I had more time to market, and my business has grown accordingly.

So, I encourage you to get rid of those barriers. Dream. Go to the top. Take that first step up the mountain. With every step you get a little higher, and the view is a little grander.

—*CLNC® Magician*

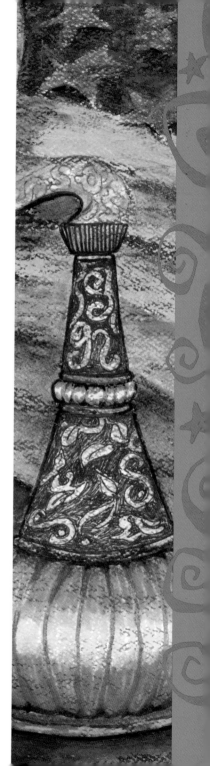

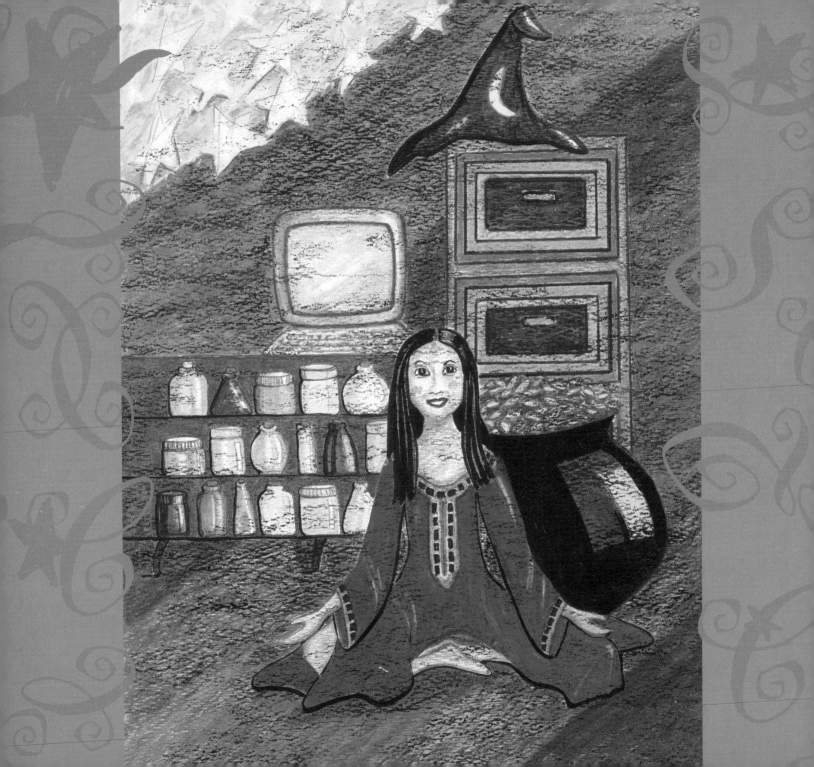

BECOME A WIZARD OF BALANCE

Your magic carpet is launched. Sales are happening. The business shows budding growth—and you need more than a Nimbus 2000 broomstick just to keep up. Balancing the magic of business development with an efficient and happy home life takes more than the twitch of your wizardly nose.

On the following pages you'll find potions for magically managing the dual challenges of business and work. You'll discover spells for gratifying self-reward and conjurations that keep you whistling through your business day while enjoying extraordinary health, effervescent energy and a positive mental attitude. You'll be your own fairy godmother. You'll move mountains. You'll enjoy a magical, mystical spirituality. With a juggler's sleight-of-hand, you'll keep a dozen balls spinning in midair while you enchant the legal world and swoop in on your broomstick to snatch golden moonbeams and become a CLNC® star.

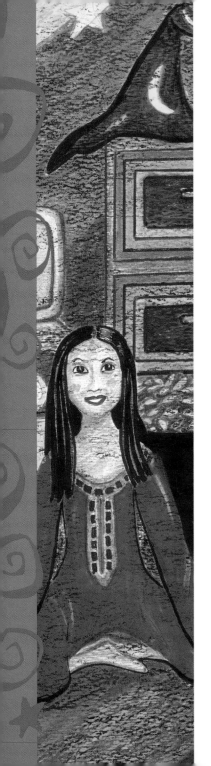

LIVE A CHARMED LIFE

You rub your magic lamp and—*poof!* The genie grants your wish for success. Suddenly you have more clients and more work coming with every ring of the phone. How do you keep your creativity at its peak? How do you continue to dazzle clients while attending to your daily incantations? Use this potion to give your wizardly right brain a regular tune-up.

Start your magic potion with:

- ✴ Energizing exercise
- ✴ Magical dietary supplements
- ✴ Sleep and relaxation
- ✴ Devilish fun
- ✴ Daily prayer or meditation
- ✴ Fascinatingly passionate work

Schedule your week to include the elements that keep you at the peak of mental, physical, emotional and spiritual health.

Surround yourself with beauty. Color, artistic line and shape stimulate the creative mind, as do rhythm, smell and sound.

Give your mind a musical massage. Totally relax for 20 minutes while playing deliciously tranquilizing music.

Luxuriate in an herbal bath while soothing your senses with aromatherapy.

Take a fun break with a playful activity at least twice a week—reading, walking on the beach, theater, ballet, a unicorn ride, a movie.

Engage in a hobby, like gardening or rock climbing, that brings you back to center.

Take time for love with your friends and family.

Treat yourself to several inspiring vacations every year.

Enjoy your work. If work ceases to be a pleasure, find a way to make it fun or find a totally new aspect of your work that you can enjoy with passion.

Appreciate your blessings. Take a daily accounting of every success, every friend and loved one, every moment of glory, small and large. Give thanks with your daily attitude of gratitude.

Genie's Tip: Do intensive mental work during your personal best time and less taxing mental work during your less productive time. Vary your activities with a few minutes of physical work followed by a period of intellectual work. Take frequent short breaks to stretch, walk, meditate, take the broomstick out for a spin or just smell the roses in your garden.

Einstein's magic moments

While lying on a hillside, dozing and contemplating the sunlight through his eyelashes, Albert Einstein made one of his important scientific discoveries. The moments just before you fall asleep, or just before you awake, are powerful and magical for conjuring new ideas or working out knotty problems that refuse to unravel during the day. Keep paper and pen at your bedside to capture these elusive images.

LEVITATE YOUR SELF-ESTEEM

Sweeping ashes out of a fireplace while her sisters flaunted their finery must have dealt a devastating blow to Cinderella's self-esteem. Then, with a swish of her fairy godmother's wand, Cinderella was wisked away to the ball, enchantingly dressed and coifed, and swept the prince right off his feet. Those fireplace cinders totally forgotten, she smiled and curtsied alongside the grandest ladies of the kingdom. When your self-esteem needs a boost, use this potion to rise above it all.

Start your magic spell with:

* Written affirmations that reaffirm what you're really good at
* A fabulous ensemble that makes you feel like a million dollars
* Uplifting music
* An affirming, upbeat friend

Optional elixir:

A makeover—hair, clothes, shoes, makeup, the works

Treat yourself regularly to an inexpensive luxury item such as a favorite chocolate, a rich-tasting wine, a massage, a manicure or pedicure.

Always have a manicured look. No matter what else is going on, take time to look good and you will automatically feel better about yourself.

Say "thank you" to compliments and relish them. Never brush aside an uplifting comment. Let your brain soak up that message.

Compliment yourself. Acknowledge your brilliance, attractiveness and dedication every time you look in the mirror, finish a work session, exercise or get a new case.

Celebrate all successes.

Magician's Tip: The brain is a phenomenal tool. It soaks up every word and expression, storing them in an emotional bank. If those words are negative—*you idiot, you clumsy fool, you slacker*—your emotional bank has only negatives on which to draw. Fill it instead with beguilingly positive statements, and your self-esteem will levitate to the clouds. Make a wizard's pact with your spouse, family member or a close friend to exchange compliments daily. Give each other at least one positive, uplifting statement every day to store in your emotional banks—*you look stunning, you're so smart, you're amazing, you're enchanting, you're Cinderella at the ball.*

A SAMPLE SPELL THAT WORKS MAGIC

Print your affirmations on your favorite note cards and post them on your bathroom mirror, in your car, near your computer, inside the kitchen cupboard, inside your luggage, beside the telephone—anywhere you might need a reminder to levitate your self-esteem.

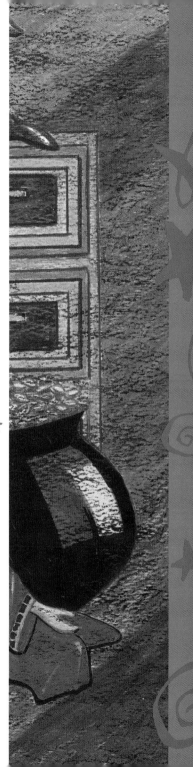

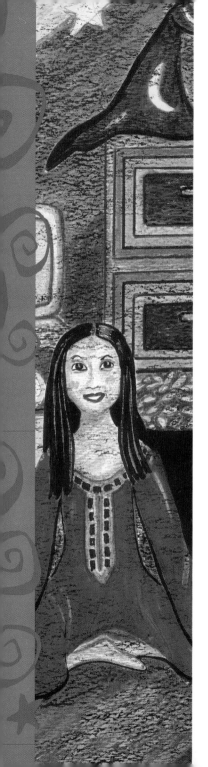

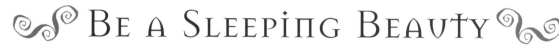

BE A SLEEPING BEAUTY

Sleep makes its own magic. It's a mood enhancer, a stress reducer, a brain-power booster. After the Sandman casts his spell, problems that seemed insurmountable during your hectic day find resolution. Life's mystifying irritations find you more tolerant. A good night's rest— seven to eight hours is the magic number—fills you with energy for tomorrow's achievements.

CONJURE AN ENCHANTING SLEEP SANCTUARY:

✳ An invitingly comfortable bed with fresh, beautiful sheets

✳ A great pillow

✳ Darkness

✳ Hypnotic music, white noise, or silence—your preference

✳ A relaxing ambience, with no work in sight

✳ A cool temperature, 70 degrees or less

OPTIONAL ELIXIR:

A warm bath, with or without bubbles, candles, a good book, a meditation CD, aromatherapy, ear plugs, sleep mask

Add your mystical rituals.

Begin your wind-down routine at the same time every night.

Wear sensual, comfortable sleepwear, or wear nothing at all.

Drink a non-caffeinated, nonalcoholic beverage.

Place a glass of water on your night table.

Remind yourself to relax at each step of your ritual.

Banish all thoughts of work or worry.

Turn out the light and sleep.

Sorcerer's Secret: Early-in-the-day exercise is a wonder-working ingredient, but avoid vigorous exercise and any thought-provoking task just before bedtime. Keep the TV, the computer and all work-related objects or papers out of your sleep sanctuary. A good night's rest is better than *abracadabra* for invoking a productive day.

BEWITCHING BEDTIME BREW

*Steep one teaspoon dried fennel in six ounces of boiling water.
Stir in one teaspoon honey, ¼ teaspoon butter and ¼ cup milk.
Banish the pixies and elves and sip your fennel tea
while listening to magically soothing music.*

TREASURE YOUR DIAMONDS, GOLD AND GYMS

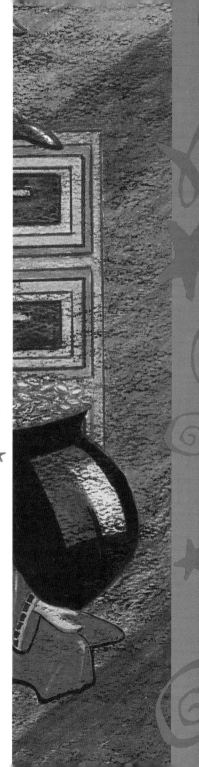

Bubble, bubble, toil and trouble—trouble is what we get when we don't exercise. Sleeplessness, lack of energy, mental sluggishness, weight gain. Invoke the incantation that will levitate you from your favorite chair and into the exercise gym. Even a brisk 20-minute walk each day will put the twinkle of gems in your eyes. Find the right exercise elixir and unmuddle your thoughts to give yourself hours more productive time. Somewhere inside of you is your fairy godmother who whispers in your ear—*"do it now!"* The trick is listening.

INVOKE YOUR OWN EXERCISE GENIE:

* Several sports you enjoy
* A time of day—no excuses, no substitutions
* A favorite environment—the park or the mall, a home gym, an exercise club, a simple exercise mat that you can slide under your bed
* A favorite workout tune—your mantra to invoke your exercise genie

OPTIONAL ELIXIR:

A personal trainer, a workout DVD, a workout partner

Engage in artful trickery. Any good sorcerer knows that proper clothing can cast its own spell, like dancing shoes make you want to tap your toes. The simple act of donning your favorite exercise clothes can entice you to work out.

Put on a good pair of sneakers or athletic shoes. Wear sensible but sensuous attire, flexible for comfort and formfitting for body awareness.

Stir in a soothsayer's common sense. Start small and listen to your body. Choose appropriate exercise for your age and health that includes stretching, aerobics and weight training.

Set goals for duration and intensity, with milestones to keep you motivated. Keep a record and reward yourself for achieving certain milestones. And don't be afraid to sweat.

Weigh in frequently to avoid illusions.

When you make exercise a habit, results will materialize like a genie from a bottle.

Do it now!

> **Wizard's Tip:** Exercise doesn't have to be boring. Add variety. Canoeing, biking, hiking, yoga, dancing and broomstick riding will each work its own magic on your body.

VICKIE'S PERSONAL WORKOUT ROUTINE

My physical fitness is the ultimate enchantment, providing the energy to keep those plates of life spinning. I do 45 minutes of weights 3 times per week, 3 to 5 aerobic sessions per week (30 to 45 minutes each) and 2 yoga sessions per week. Additionally, most of our vacations are biking or hiking trips. I love to eat and this routine allows me to! I perform this magic spell first thing in the morning so nothing can jinx my day.

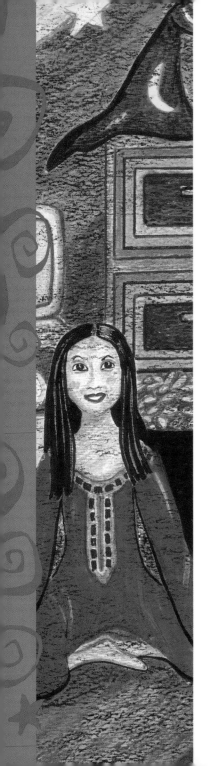

Buzz Around with the Extraordinary Energy of Vickie and Tinkerbell

The average gnome lives 600 years. Elves, fairies and selected immortal wizards live forever. With excellent health you can expect to enjoy such longevity and have plenty of energy for your business. When your health fails, or is even off just slightly, no pixie dust, hoodoo or white magic will work its spell. How do you keep up? Where do you get the energy to sprinkle pixie dust on all your projects? Do what Tinkerbell and I do. Cast this spell daily.

Start your magic spell with:

✦ 7 to 8 hours of restful sleep per night—not per week

✦ A healthy protein shake or one of the ingredients from Vickie's Personal Prescription

✦ 10 minutes of quiet time to plan your day

Begin each day by taking the time to plan for balance. The first incantation you cast each morning should be a spell-weaving ritual that attracts the fairies of fitness and keeps you extraordinarily energized. Your mind, body and soul all need attention. Excellent health comes from stirring in a measure of each.

Engage in a scheduled exercise routine at least one hour five days a week.

Eat energizing meals. Eat small quantities of healthy, low-sugar foods every four hours. Indulge in occasional favorite treats like popcorn at the Quiddich game. Take vitamins and antioxidants daily, and enjoy special wizards' treats: flaxseed and green tea.

Share food preparation with your spouse and kids.

Keep your regular medical check-ups.

Pamper yourself occasionally. Schedule empty time for spontaneous walks, baths, a movie, a good novel and personal hobbies.

Find a reason to laugh every single day.

Enchanting Extras

• A sprinkle of laughter.

• A dash of spiritual growth time.

• A phone visit with a friend.

• A romantic date night out.

• A massage.

• A manicure, pedicure, facial or hair salon appointment.

• A leisurely bath, with bubbles, candles, music and a favorite drink.

• 30 minutes of personal time to indulge in a fun project or simply nothing important.

• A daily meditation moment.

VICKIE'S PERSONAL PRESCRIPTION FOR OPTIMAL HEALTH

- Exercise—my goal is to exercise at least five days a week. I love hiking, yoga, Pilates, biking and working with weights.

- Massage—a once-a-week massage renews my energy.

- Vacation—I schedule 12 weeks of vacation for myself every year.

- Time with spouse and family—time for love. In a herd of elephants, when one falls the others pick him up. I love being surrounded by my own family of elephants.

- Daily prayer and meditation—I'm most creative in the silence.

- Weight control—I eat mostly healthy low-sugar foods and lots of veggies and protein.

- Supplements—flaxseed, green tea, vitamins and antioxidants are part of my daily regimen.

- Fun—I schedule something fun at least twice a week, including time for things I love—reading, walks with my husband, our whirlpool, theater and musicals.

- Sleep—I get seven to eight hours sleep per night.

- Taking Sunday off—I don't even make my bed.

- Working my passion—I revolutionize nursing careers one RN at a time.

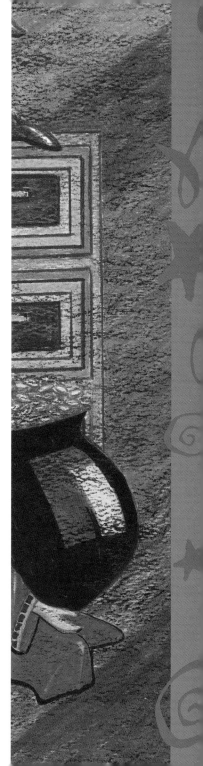

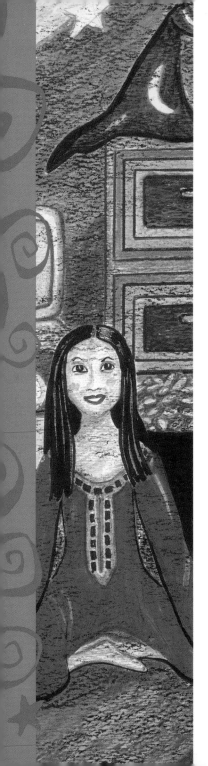

Connect with Your Magical Spirituality

Enchantment lies where spirit and instinct are in true harmony. When you feel as if you're turning into stone, there is no evil hex that a few moments alone with your spirituality cannot neutralize or perhaps even transform into positive energy. Whether you call it prayer, meditation or simply quiet time, your true path will materialize when you connect daily with spiritual guidance.

Conjure an Ethereal Atmosphere:

✴ A spiritual sanctuary, physical or mental
✴ A spiritual book
✴ Spiritual quotes or affirmations
✴ Spiritual music

Optional Elixir:

A cross, rosary or other spiritual symbol

Compose your spiritual moment in the sanctity of your own mind. Read a scripture or a passage from a book on positive thinking or a book of poetry. Appreciate beauty in simplicity. Be happy with who you are. Look within and discover peace.

Shaman's Secret: Five minutes of quiet time every two hours can renew you more powerfully than a half-hour nap. Consider spending this special time outdoors. A nearness to nature keeps the spirit sensitive to impressions not commonly felt and in touch with unseen powers.

Spirituality is an Individual Choice

Prayer for Protection

The light of God surrounds me;

The love of God enfolds me;

The power of God protects me;

The presence of God watches over me.

Wherever I am, God is!

—*from the Unity Church of Christianity*

Whistle While You Work

Since you spend at least half of your waking hours working, doesn't it make sense for that work to be fun? It takes only a little wizardry to stave off the trolls of tedium and ensure an impishly playful life as a CLNC® consultant.

Assemble your wizard's workshop:

* An enchanting, personalized office environment
* A terrific view or a fabulous painting
* A treasure chest of treats on your desk
* Energizing music

Optional elixir:

A fanciful screensaver, a humorous calendar

Stir your bewitching workday with:

✓ People who make you happy. Surround yourself with associates, employees, vendors and salespeople you enjoy. Become a mentor to someone you appreciate. Fire difficult clients.

✓ A change of pace. Take a brainstorming walk, alone or with another wizard. Work outside for a while. Appropriate a table in your favorite coffee shop.

✓ Frequent rewards. Sneak away to an early movie after working on a difficult project.

✓ Something new for yourself or your business. Choose from a prepared reward list. Or simply enjoy a glass of wine or a special treat at the end of each workday.

Finish the following sentence and look at it daily.

What I love most about my CLNC® business is

_____

_____

_____

Sorcerer's Secret Ingredient: Joy. Take your business seriously, but don't take yourself seriously. Give yourself permission to make a mistake. Look for the humor in every situation, and with a flourish of your wand, turn your business into a magical adventure. The reward is well worth the effort.

Personalize your wizard's work space

In addition to photographs of family and friends, include pictures of people who inspire you, fresh flowers or plants, scented candles, inspirational posters, poetry or quotations, toys or a devilishly quick game you can enjoy during break time.

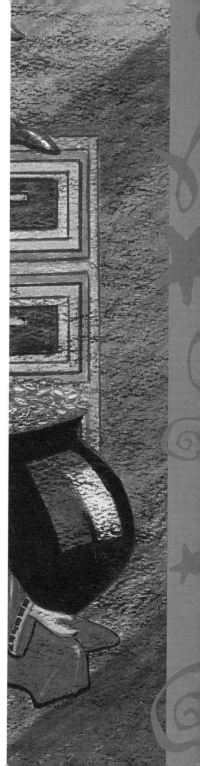

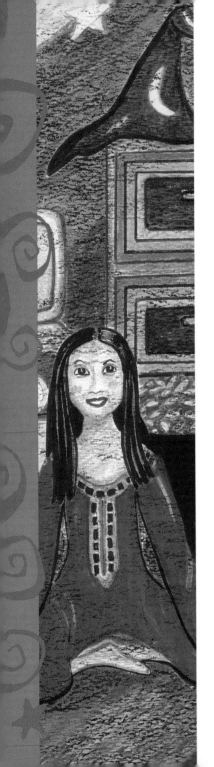

Juggle Your Work and Family

An accomplished magician is a master of balance—spinning plates, juggling fire and knowing precisely how to saw the lady in half. The jugglery of a Certified Legal Nurse Consultant^{CM} involves commitment to maintaining a healthy, happy, accommodating family while growing a successful CLNC® business. Invoke this magic spell to keep those plates spinning.

Start your incantation with:

* A designated work space with a door
* A scheduled work day with a definite beginning and end
* One day devoted to family—no work allowed
* A separate business phone

Optional elixir:

A special game or activity, like Quiddich or wizard's chess, that you all enjoy together

Keep the promises you make to your family. Post the family calendar where everyone can see it and highlight family events on your personal calendar.

Make a priority of eating meals together as a family.

Prepare food together. Give each family member a fun part of conjuring the meal as well as a clean-up task.

Hire outside help for household chores or make the chores a family event.

Schedule quiet reading times—sharing a space in silence. Work together but on different things for example, kids doing homework, while you write a report.

Take mini-adventures with your family while another wizard covers for you.

Schedule date nights.

My next family adventure is

_____

_____

Soothsayer's Advice: Involve your entire family in your business planning and let them know how much you value their support. Let them help you spin those plates. Take a family member along on a business trip. Delegate a business task to each child—with pay. A wizard's kids can copy, staple, fax, label or file. A sorcerer's spouse might be in charge of billing or updating your mailing list or something he or she does well.

A sample spell that works magic

When it's time to mail out your information newsletter, rustle up some popcorn and pop in a movie while everyone folds, staples and stamps. Then load the family on the broomstick to head for the post office. When you receive that first response, announce it to the whole family and celebrate.

Cast 2 Spells at Once

To grow your business and your kids at the same time, you must be part wizard, part shaman, part clairvoyant. Your day begins earlier and ends later than anyone else's. You bandage a skinned knee with one hand while answering a client's call with the other. Working at home, you have the joy as well as the headaches of spending more time with your family. The trick is in knowing when to sprinkle a bit of pixie dust and when to lay on a real hex.

Conjure a supporting environment:

✷ An office with a door
✷ A game room or playroom for the kids

Mystic rules for:

- Entering the office
- Not answering the phone
- Keeping spaghetti sauce off paperwork
- Using the copy machine
- Designating and sharing chores
- Having a clear definition of "emergency"
- Scheduling meals and treats
- Caring for pets
- Spending time outdoors

Optional elixir:

A housekeeper, nanny, babysitter, fairy godmother, kid's day out

Stir in bushels of patience and humor, a supportive spouse or friend, and a dash of flexibility.

Schedule frequent breaks to check on what's happening and quality time for shared hobbies.

Trade dinner nights out with your spouse and teenagers.

Enlist your children's help with filing, sorting, copying and mailing.

Keep preschoolers in sight. Give them a magic legal pad to draw on and a secret signal for break time.

> **Fortune-Teller's Insight:** Working and raising kids can be as rewarding as you make it. The most important ingredient is a clear sense of priorities. Have a back-up plan for handling the unexpected and a reward system for the whole family.

The Kid's Home Office

Why not set up an office for your kids? Cathy Bakalar's success story might give you some ideas. While Cathy focused on her business, her daughters asked questions such as, "What is a mission statement?" or "How many pages does a business plan need to be?" Cathy answered their questions and shooed them off to play while she worked nonstop for several weeks.

While tidying the girls' playroom, she noticed signs taped to their chairs. The signs read President, Vice President and Secretary. She found a binder labeled "Kitten Sittin'." Inside the binder was a mission statement, a business plan and ideas for business cards. One card read: "21 years of kitten sitting experience." They and a friend were starting their own business.

Six months later, the girls had earned over $100.00. Now their income projection posters for the next year proudly hang on the wall in their "office."

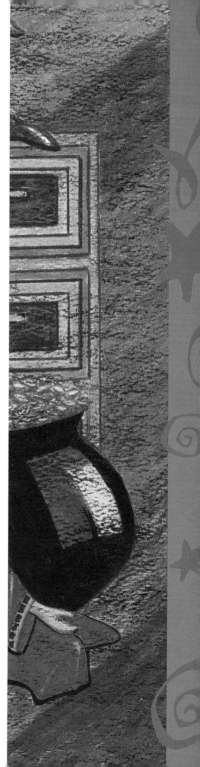

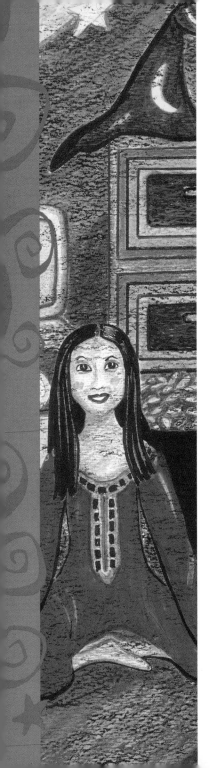

PLAN AN ENCHANTING VACATION

The ultimate elixir for mind, body and soul is a getaway. Is your dream vacation a romantic adventure? A fun-filled frolic with your family? A solitary stroll through an exotic city? Take that magical time away from your ordinary world and you will rechannel your energy to higher levels of CLNC® success. Don't let vacation time vanish in a flurry of activity that leaves you more exhausted than when you left. Conjure the perfect getaway.

ASSEMBLE YOUR ALCHEMIST'S TOOLS:

* A globe or a map
* Travel brochures, travel books, travel DVDs
* A calendar
* A sense of adventure
* A whimsical attitude
* A well-traveled friend

OPTIONAL ELIXIR:

A travel planner, travel companions, a magic carpet

Prepare for your creative adventure by paging through the books and brochures, watching the DVDs, visiting the Internet for airline prices, hotel arrangements and additional information about exciting locales.

Seek travel ideas from other well-traveled friends.

Make a wish list of five dream vacations.

Mix in a little clairvoyance, a vision of wonders you might encounter, an expectation of exciting moments, exotic foods you might enjoy.

Then mark the date and destination on your calendar.

MY NEXT VACATION IS

_____

_____

_____

Soothsayer's Suggestion: Schedule your vacations each year *before* you schedule anything else—and *take them.* Clear your work calendar, tie up loose ends with clients, get a CLNC® wizard to cover for you, and when you go, *be* on vacation. Don't allow work to enter your mind. Explore new places and try new things, but also allow some serenity to appreciate your experiences. Enjoy, relax and you'll return enchantingly refreshed.

ENHANCE YOUR VACATION WITH

* A good book to read on the airplane
* A camera and travel journal to record your experiences
* Sheet protectors in a 3-ring binder for travel brochures and mementoes you collect
* An adventurous attitude

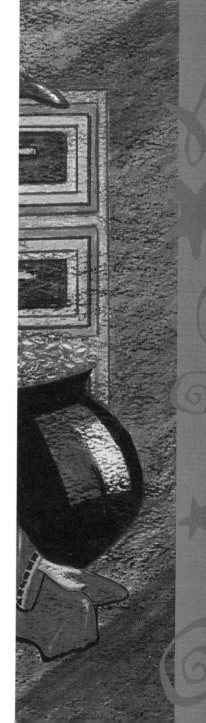

My perfect getaways
(Or my 5 dream vacations)

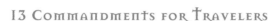

_____

_____

_____

_____

_____

13 Commandments for Travelers

1. Thou shalt not expect to find things as thou has left them at home, for thou hast left home to find things different.

2. Thou shalt not take anything too seriously, for a carefree mind is the beginning of an excellent vacation.

3. Thou shalt not let other tourists get on thy nerves, for thou art paying good money to have a good time.

4. Remember thy passport so that thou knowest where it is at all times, for a person without a passport is a person without a country.

5. Blessed is the person who can say "thank you" in any language.

6. Make up thy mind to be happy, for thou can think thyself into being miserable. Learn to find pleasure in simple things.

7. Thou shalt not worry, for he who worrieth has no pleasure, and few things are ever fatal.

8. Thou shalt not judge the people of a country by one person with whom thou has had difficulty.

9. Thou shalt, when in Rome, do as the Romans do; if in difficulty, thou shalt use thy common sense and friendliness.

10. Remember, thou art a guest in every land, and he who treateth his host with respect shall be treated as an honored guest.

11. Remember, if thou were created to stay in one place, thou would have grown roots.

12. Whilst thou art away, look around and realize how lucky thou art at home.

13. As Erma Bombeck sayeth, "When thou looks like thy passport photo, it's time to returneth home."

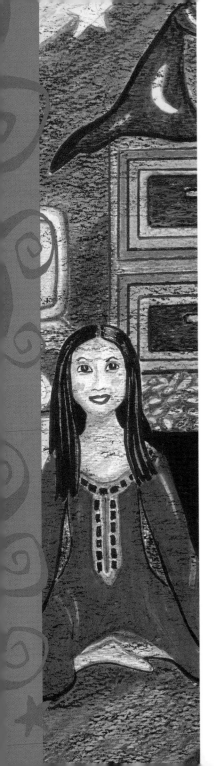

BE YOUR OWN FAIRY GODMOTHER

L ike leaving out treats to reward the gnomes, fairies and little people who bring us luck, the best way to ensure that success repeats itself is to acknowledge and celebrate each occurrence. Take a moment to bask in the glow of completing a successful project. Call a friend or associate to share the thrill. Choose a reward and enjoy it.

Start your reward incantation with:

* A guilt-free commitment to "do it"
* A song that reflects your glory and excitement
* Plenty of time for reflection
* Your *I Am a Successful CLNC® Success Journal*

Optional elixir:

A spouse, friend or family member to help you celebrate

Prepare yourself for success by creating and enjoying a list of your favorite rewards.

- A cultural event—theater, museum, ballet, concert
- An unscheduled celebration day off
- A weekend getaway
- A matinee movie
- A spa treatment
- A nature walk

- Dinner out
- Flowers or chocolates
- An expensive new business suit, briefcase or accessory
- Time for yourself—to sleep in, go dancing, read a book

My next reward is

_____

_____

Wizard's Tip: Don't wait to celebrate your arrival at the big success. Celebrate milestones along the way. Use your *CLNC® Success Journal* to record each rewarding juncture and read it often. Save congratulatory letters and cards to read when the road gets particularly rough. Select a symbolic reminder that you are a talented, resourceful CLNC® consultant—a song that makes you happy, a charm such as an enchanting piece of jewelry or perhaps a picture of a favorite elf.

Celebrate your milestones

CLNC® Certification achieved, completed promotional package, first interview, first case, first check, first case completed, clinical salary matched, first $10,000.00, full-time CLNC® status, first year in business, a business challenge conquered, clinical salary doubled.

Move Mountains with Positive Thinking

When Sleeping Beauty was born, three charming fairies brought the gifts of happiness, beauty and laughter. Then a fourth fairy, Maleficent, appeared, uninvited. *"Where you go the shadow of sorrow follows,"* the king told Maleficent. Have you ever noticed that some people bring shadows and negativity into every situation? They are beaten before they start. Your ability to move mountains begins with one magical phrase, *"I can."*

Begin your potion with:

* A commitment to positive thinking
* A list of friends and family who bring positive influence into your life
* Hypnotically positive affirmations such as "I can"
* A ready smile

Optional elixir:

The children's book, *The Little Engine That Could* **by Watty Piper**

Become aware of your negative thoughts. If you catch yourself thinking, *"I haven't a clue how to write this report,"* change that to a positive thought, *"I have the nursing experience and CLNC® know-how to write a great report."*

Keep stirring your potion, adding your personal values, passions and dreams.

Limit your exposure to negative influences. Hang with winners, not whiners. Surround yourself with powerful positive forces.

Devise a plan of transfiguration and decide to begin thinking in a positive manner. Read books and listen to CDs on the power of positive thinking. Smile often.

Recite positive affirmations when going to an interview, starting a project, writing your first report, when a dragon client roars or when negative thoughts threaten to surface.

> **Fortune-Teller's Tip:** When you focus on what's wrong, you cannot see what's possible. If you're concentrating on the problems, you'll never see the opportunities. If you see a glass as half empty, think of the potential to fill it up. Anything is possible— just determine how badly you want it and murmur the magic words, *"I can."*

Sample affirmations that work magic

* I have what it takes to succeed.
* I have the energy to make this happen.
* I love learning new things every day.
* I'm a bright, intelligent, talented, determined and powerful CLNC® wizard.
* Every day in every way I get better and better.
* I'm a successful CLNC® consultant.
* I'm a nurse. I can do anything.

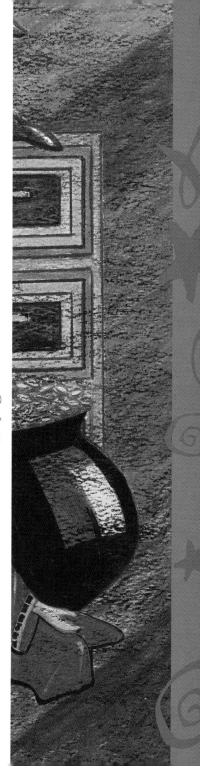

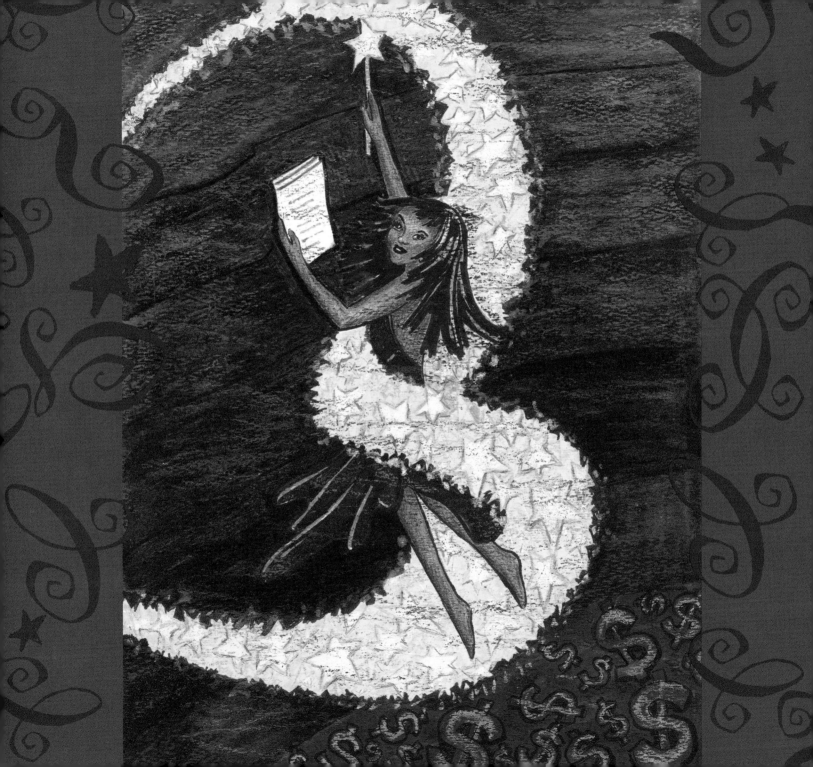

ADD EXTRA SPARKLE TO YOUR CLNC® WIZARDRY

Beyond the ordinary lies Xanadu, Utopia, Shangri'la—the best of all possible worlds, where dreams, vision and imagination become reality. Only the most dedicated of wizards will reach this ideal. Those willing to go that extra mile, to reach beyond the stars and boldly fly toward the air castle of their vision will make excellent use of the hexes and potions that follow.

The magic of mighty alliances, perceptive mentors and gratitude—these are the finishing strokes that turn neophytes into master magicians. Use them wisely. A flourish of the wand and your dream world unfolds in a cascade of brilliance.

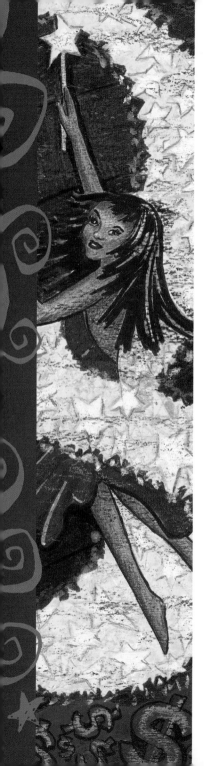

Sprinkle Attitude-of-Gratitude Fairy Dust All Over the World

Any good wizard knows that amassing positive energy enhances a spell's power. Gratitude is a powerful elixir. Be grateful for your success, and—*alakazam!*—a magic portal will open to more and bigger successes.

Start your magic spell with:

* Your philosophy of life
* Your vision statement
* A favorite thought, feeling or experience
* Note cards for expressing thanks, congratulations and other good thoughts
* A commitment to expressing thanks a dozen times a day
* Small gifts and flowers

Optional elixir:

A prayer or meditation

Invoke white magic by recognizing someone else's contribution to your success.

* Send frequent notes, emails and voice mails of appreciation to your attorney-clients and their staff.
* Create a gratitude journal. Use photos and words to express appreciation for each milestone.

* Adopt an elf, gnome or angel whose depiction symbolizes thanks.
* Write down what your CLNC® business has done for you, what you get from your business, why you wake up grateful each day and go eagerly to work.
* Share your magic with a friend. Bring a smile to a dozen faces. Commit random acts of kindness.
* Acknowledge one thing you're grateful for before you fall asleep at night and when you awaken each morning.

> **Wizard's Tip:** The heart of your CLNC® business is an attitude of gratitude. Maintain a sense of humor and appreciation regardless of what's happening around you. Never RSVP to your own pity party. Be willing to work with the situation at hand and expect spectacular results. Look for goodness and you'll find goodness. A sprinkle of good-fairy dust works wonders.

Instances when you might need this spell

* When a project turns out better than expected.
* When a project turns sour.

Entertain with Captivating Elegance

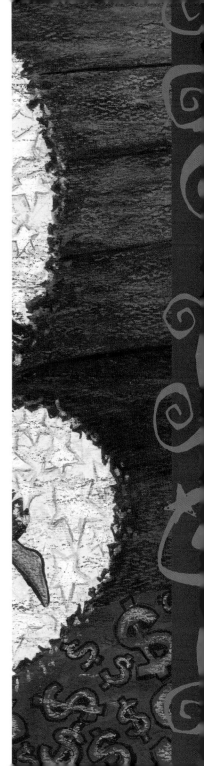

usiness entertaining is an opportunity to connect with attorney-prospects and clients on neutral ground and in a relaxed atmosphere. Have fun, build rapport and get to know each other while maintaining a professional demeanor. The easy magic of clever planning and proper etiquette can save you from the sort of havoc Alice encountered at the Mad Hatter's Tea Party.

Start your magic spell with:

* The appropriate business attire—leave your wizard's robe at home
* A credit card
* A reserved table
* A list of six conversation starters

Optional elixir:

Business Etiquette in Brief: The Competitive Edge for Today's Professional by Ann Marie Sabath, or the *Prentice Hall Complete Business Etiquette Handbook* by Barbara Pachter, Betsy Anderson and Marjorie Brody

Match the restaurant to the attorney. Ask the attorney's secretary for the name of the attorney's favorite but rarely frequented restaurant.

Communicate in advance that you are the host. Reserve your preferred table—away from the bathroom, kitchen or water station—and arrange to receive the bill.

Check in 15 minutes early. Turn off your cell phone as soon as your client arrives and won't be trying to call to say she's been delayed.

Follow the attorney's lead. If he skips an appetizer, do likewise. Avoid food that has a high potential for causing accidents.

Respect the attorney's time. Don't turn a one-hour lunch into two hours.

Make your follow-up thank-you note appear almost instantly in your guest's mailbox.

> **Soothsayer's Advice:** Entertain at breakfast—where you will strain to run up a serious tab. This also eliminates the issue of drinking alcohol. Above all, don't let worrying about appropriate etiquette or any awkward situation keep you from enjoying your guest and making the most of your business occasion. Keep a sorcerer's sense of humor.

Dining etiquette

Fortunately, you can practice the wizardly use of utensils, place settings and manners in the comfort of your own castle before you engage in your first business dining experience. The basics are easy:

* Touch your index fingers to your thumbs. Your left hand forms a "b" for bread and your right hand forms a "d" for drink. Your bread plate is on the left of the dinner plate and your drinks always go on the right.
* Begin with the utensils farthest from the plate on either side. A utensil placed above the plate is used for dessert.
* Offer dinner rolls, salad dressings and other food items to your guests before helping yourself. Present the item to the person on your left first, then pass it to your right.

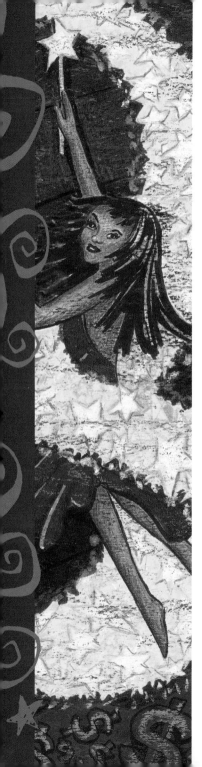

GET STRONGER WITH EVERY SPELL

"Opportunity is missed by most people because it is dressed in overalls and looks like work."
—*Thomas A. Edison*

A wizard's powers increase with experience and practice. Never let a day go by that you don't conjure at least one easy spell. Among the variety in this book you'll find conjurations for your busiest as well as your most leisurely days. Use them frequently to keep your sorcery skills sharp and your CLNC® business acumen strong.

Start your incantation with:

* A pair of five-pound dumbbells
* One strength-building exercise
* Your *I Am a Successful CLNC® Success Journal*
* A list of friends who are there for you
* Photos of three people you can really depend on

Start every spell by briefly reviewing your preferred outcome, the essential ingredients and the step-by-step order of achievement.

Prime your mental and emotional pump with affirmations. Envision a person you admire egging you on with supportive statements.

Proceed with confidence and enthusiasm.

Review the results, noting what went well and where you might improve.

Celebrate every success, no matter how minor.

Record in your journal every crisis, loss and disappointment, as well as every accomplishment, triumph, fortune and joy.

Celebrate with other CLNC® consultants.

> **Wizard's Tip:** Remember, an easy life and a good life are not the same thing. Adopt a hobby that makes you feel stronger. Success in your avocation strengthens your ability and resolve in other areas. Cultivate the fire of desire and choose an active, physically challenging hobby. The day-to-day work of a CLNC® consultant is generally cerebral and sedentary, constantly taxing and toning the brain while neglecting the body. You need to keep your physical muscles in tone for whalloping unreasonable dragons.

The Serenity Prayer

Grant me the serenity to accept the things I cannot change, courage to change the things I can, and the wisdom to know the difference.

Living one day at a time; enjoying one moment at a time; accepting hardship as the pathway to peace. Taking this...world as it is, not as I would have it. Trusting that He will make all things right if I surrender to His will; that I may be reasonably happy in this life, and supremely happy forever in the next.

—*Rev. Reinhold Neibuhr*

Harness the Force with Mighty Alliances

There is strength in numbers and magic in the number three. Two people create opposing forces, a third creates balance. Align with two other CLNC® wizards and you can accomplish the most complicated spell or brew up the most elusive potion.

Start your magic spell with:

* A list of people you admire
* A list of professionals you like to work with—banker, artist, writer
* A list of Certified Legal Nurse Consultants[CM] with whom you would like to align
* A list of community and social events where you will meet professionals from other industries

Optional elixir:

Think and Grow Rich by **Napoleon Hill**

Systemize networking and brainstorming with professional business owners who are not CLNC® consultants at least once a month.

Join a serious executive or CEO group that will be your informal board of advisors.

Establish a mastermind relationship with two CLNC® consultants who are outside your geographical area.

Agree on a regular date and time to mastermind on specific objectives.

Stick to your allotted time.

Agree to share other alliance activities, such as locating expert witnesses and covering for each other PRN.

Show an attitude of gratitude. Be careful not to overstep boundaries—you are all equal but with different areas of expertise, knowledge and experience.

After three months, evaluate how well your mastermind group is working and change as necessary.

My mastermind group includes

_____

_____

_____

Wizard's Tip: Participate in *National Alliance of Certified Legal Nurse Consultants'* activities, such as the annual *NACLNC®* Conference.

"I go forth alone and stand as 10,000."
— *Maya Angelou*

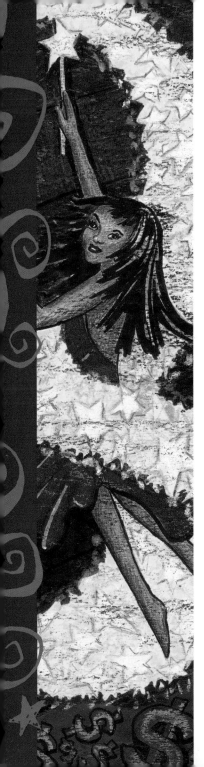

Use the Institute's CLNC® Mentors Like a True Magician

"The great Oz knows all," Dorothy thought. Yet the Lion already had his courage, the Tin Man already had a heart and the Scarecrow already had a brain. The great wizard only pointed out what they already knew. Many times this is exactly what happens between you and your CLNC® Mentor. Perhaps you already have the answers but don't yet have the confidence to trust your instincts. Use this spell to guide you in using the Institute's free mentoring services.

Start your magic mentoring potion with:

★ The CLNC® Certification Program

You'll find the Institute's online Mentoring Request Form in the *NACLNC®* Community.

Use the CLNC® Mentoring Program as a resource, and opportunity to grow.

Challenge yourself. Write your own resume, create your own marketing plan and grow your own business. The Institute will help you brainstorm ideas, will review your legal nurse consulting and business practices, and will help you face each new challenge with confidence.

Follow the step-by-step potion:

- Capture your issue or challenge in writing.
- Outline your overall goal and the desired outcome.
- Identify the strategies you have already implemented to solve your issue or challenge.

- Refer to your CLNC® educational resources to sharpen your problem-solving skills.
- Complete the Institute's online Mentoring Request Form which you'll find in the *NACLNC®* Community.

When you access the Institute's mentors, you will be matched with a CLNC® Mentor who has special knowledge in the area where you have questions.

Just as Merlin saw the makings of a king in Arthur, the CLNC® Mentor will recognize your strengths and will coach to those strengths. Your special Merlin will set you back on course when you feel lost, will help you envision your next step and will hold you accountable for performance when you long to make a quick conjuration and be done. Mentoring advice from the CLNC® wizard will save you from hundreds of failed spells.

> **Wizard's Tip:** As Merlin said to Arthur in D.H. White's *The Once and Future King,* "The only thing that will always make you feel good is to learn something new." The purpose of the Institute's mentoring program is not to make your decisions for you but to guide you toward making better decisions on your own. The CLNC® Mentor is a wise and trusted counselor, not a therapist.

7 Tips to Tapping the Magic of a Magus

1. Think through the issue yourself before requesting mentoring.
2. Always be organized and respectful.
3. Take notes.
4. Act immediately on the advice you receive.
5. Take responsibility for your actions and the success of your business.
6. When you succeed, share the glory. Acknowledge the help you received.

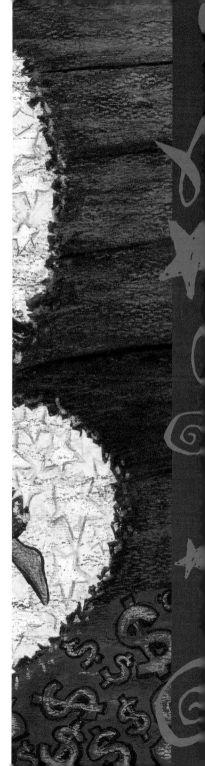

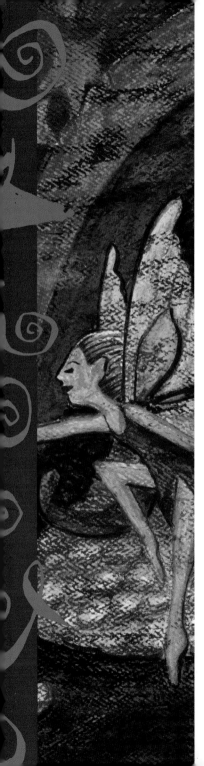

OTHER LEGAL NURSE CONSULTING RESOURCES
FROM VICKIE MILAZZO INSTITUTE

Basic CLNC® Certification Program
Taught by the pioneer of legal nurse consulting, Vickie L. Milazzo, the author of the *Core Curriculum for Legal Nurse Consulting*® textbook. Get certified in only 6 days—Home-Study (DVD or CD) or Seminar.

Medical-Related Case Reports
Vickie and the CLNC® Pros share actual reports submitted to attorneys. They show you how to write superb reports that will win you repeat business for your CLNC® practice.

Advanced CLNC® Practice-Building Programs
Quickly grow your CLNC® practice with this advanced collection of powerful, time-tested tools and techniques.

- The Power of CLNC® Focus
- The Secret Life of a CLNC® Entrepreneur
- Winning Relationships—Your Jackpot for CLNC® Success

NACLNC® Apprenticeship
You'll master report writing strategies and develop your 90-day marketing plan. Roll up your sleeves and apply the skills you learned in the CLNC® Certification Program. Available on Home-Study (DVD or CD) or 2-Day Live.

CLNC® Marketing LaunchBox
Launch your CLNC® practice with this complete start-up marketing package. Your CLNC® Marketing LaunchBox saves you thousands of dollars *Plus* you're ready to start marketing to attorneys immediately. You don't have to spend time and money on the tedious task of putting your marketing packet together on your own. Our expert copywriters and professional designers have done it for you.

Private *NACLNC*® Apprenticeship
Be one of only seven apprentices to live a week in the life of a full-time practicing CLNC® Mentor.

You will work on real cases and projects in a live environment and master the strategies of running a successful and efficient CLNC® practice from a home office.

Flash 55 Free Promotions—55 FREE Ways to Promote Your CLNC® Business, Second Edition
Market your CLNC® practice FREE with these 55 fast, easy ideas.

Success Journal—I Am a Successful CLNC®
With Vickie's favorite quotes and success steps, this journal will help you capture and relive your extraordinary CLNC® journey. Includes the first 25 steps for launching your CLNC® business.

e-Contracts! Contracts! Contracts!
The only CLNC® contracts you'll ever need. Ten customizable contracts *PLUS* a FREE contracts e-textbook. Personalize, print and go.

Inside Every Woman: Using the 10 Strengths You Didn't Know You Had to Get the Career and Life You Want Now
In this energizing and eye-opening *Wall Street Journal* bestseller, Vickie openly discusses the obstacles she and other women overcame on their paths to success. She shows you how to amplify your strengths with laser-like focus and make simple adjustments that will help you achieve the career you want and the life you desire. Also, available in DVD and audio CD.

NACLNC® Community
Exclusive online resources for *NACLNC®* members only.

Legal Nurse Consulting Ezine Archive at LNCEzine.com
This extensive archive includes hundreds of articles, tips and best practices from Vickie Milazzo and the CLNC® Pros.

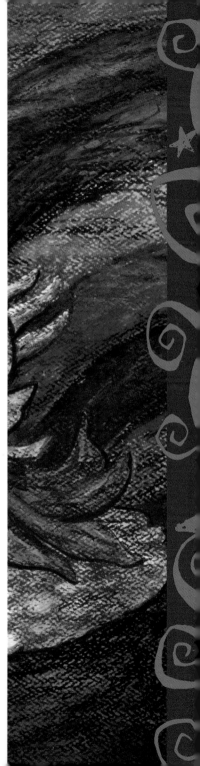